ihl

incredible

healing

library

3

BOOKS BY LISA ROBBINS
The Cancer Journal Heal Yourself!

BOOKS CO-AUTHORED BY LISA ROBBINS
The Power of 100
12 Letters To The Women Of The World

COURSES BY LISA ROBBINS
The 10 Key Principles of Healing Transformational
Experience

Meet Lisa online and access free
teaching, cleanses and healing recipes at
www.TheGoodWitch.ca

Watch inspiring cure and survivor stories of many
different 'dis-eases' at
www.IncredibleHealingJournals.com

Learn how to cleanse, heal and rebuild your body
through the *10 Key Principles Of Healing*
***Transformational Experience* course of study**
www.HealingCancer.ca

Cancer Cure and Survivor Stories

How To Cure Cancer Series

Let's Talk About Healing And What Works:

Uplifting stories of how people cure themselves by moving through cancer, healing their bodies and their lives.

By:

Lisa Robbins, BScHN, RHN, CTT

Co Authors:

Evangelina Aguilar
Kapil Arn
Elaine Cantin
Yvonne Chamberlain
Brenda Cobb
Linda Devine
Dr. Sue Gelder
Pattie McDonald
Chris Wark
Nuro Weidemann

Incredible Healing Library

Ontario, Canada

ihl

Incredible Healing Library
Ontario, Canada

For information about special discounts for bulk purchases, please send an email to: BulkOrders@IncredibleHealingJournals.com

Editor: Thank You Alexandra Robbins.

Cover Design: Thank You Paul Clark.
www.wearevirtuallyeverywhere.com

Manufactured in Canada and United States

Robbins, Lisa

Cancer Cure and Survivor Stories

International Standard Book Numbers
Printed Book ISBN: 978-0-9864902-7-9
Electronic Book ISBN: 978-0-9864902-8-6
Audio Book ISBN: Forthcoming

Dedicated To You

I hope the stories in this book add to your wisdom and insight, to help carry you on your journey through 'dis-ease,' to your perfect vision of health and happiness.

With much love,

Lisa

Our Readers Say:

"I really enjoyed reading Cancer Cure and Survivor Stories. It was nice to find a variety of testimonials in one place. It shows there are many different ways to overcome cancer. I found most had a few things in common, maintain a positive attitude and do what you feel is right for your body instead of what the conventional doctors push for. I wish you luck with this and look forward to learning more from you."

Kathy Powers

"This book contains many uplifting stories about people who survived their cancer without resorting to drastic measures such as surgery, chemotherapy and/or radiation. It gives one hope there are alternative cures for cancer that work!!"

John Tod

"It took only moments to identify with some of the situations and circumstances described in the remarkably candid accounts presented here. I found myself whispering "me too," as I read through the different accounts, written by inspiring people. I also want to emphasize that the accounts presented here would bring great value to anybody who had recently been given distressing news that they had developed dis-ease which conventional medicine diagnoses as 'fatal' and gives a 'time-running-out' prognosis.

I particularly like the 'Points To Remember' lists at the end of each account – very useful on days when energy and time are scarce but you nevertheless need a quick reminder just how to stay positive and buoyant when the babbling brook of life becomes a torrent! I feel they give just enough to remind us that it can be done. They are encouraging, even if you don't have time to read through the whole account again.

Some useful recommendations are given in terms of where to start and where to go for further information. I get the feeling I will be referring to these again in future and I am thankful for that!"

Mike Dancer

Table of Contents

"All truths are easy to understand once they are discovered,
The point is to discover them."

Galileo Galilei

Disclaimer

The information in this book is for educational and information sharing purposes only. This book was written to share how others have used nutrition and natural therapies, along with medical treatments and surgical procedures, to kill and remove cancer cells and whole tumors and to heal their bodies and lives.

Some of the people whose stories are in these pages continue to move through cancer. Some do not suffer from the 'dis-ease' called cancer anymore. Some remain free from cancer, anywhere from two to more than 30 years. The people who share these stories do so to help others. In many cases, spreading the joy of healing and the way to achieve optimum health has become their life's work.

This book and the stories shared here are not a substitute for the diagnosis or treatment of disease, nor are they meant to replace the advice of a qualified practitioner.

Please consult a qualified practitioner before you use any herbal, food or natural therapy discussed in these pages to be sure it will not interfere with, enhance the activity of or render useless any prescribed medication or natural herbal product you may be taking or any condition you may be experiencing.

No author here is claiming that any health product or food or any combination thereof cures cancer. Every person and situation is different and all results are different. Please know what you are putting in and on your body and what the consequences are at all times. You shoulder the responsibility for your health and life and thankfully so, because no one cares more for you, than you.

If you do not wish to be bound by the above Disclaimer, please return this book immediately for a refund of your monies and destroy all copies, electronic and otherwise, of the printed material and audiobook, if applicable.

Greetings

It is my hope that through sharing the beautiful stories in these pages they will help you to connect with your own inner strength. We have come to see that this is the most important aspect of all.

There are many teachings in every healing journey, each one molded by the experiences and perceptions of the individual. Healing provides for an expansion of awareness, an evolution through 'dis-ease' to a healthier, happier and more peaceful way of living.

Each healing journey is unique. Some people find deep cleansing and healing in a raw diet, which throws off years of built up toxins and helps to release long-held recurring emotions. Others use the healing strength of a traditional macrobiotic diet to cleanse, heal and rebuild. Still others are focused on healing from an energetic level and desire therapies that calmly promote wellness by balancing physical vibration and energy flow.

Whatever therapy, diet or state of mind used to bring healing, the golden thread that weaves its way through these stories is a deep desire to live, fortified with an eager willingness to do everything possible.

My wish for you is that no matter what place you are in right now, you are able to grow your strength into a powerful force to heal your body and your life.

With much love and hope for a healthy, happy future.

Lisa

oxo

1   Tap Into Your Inner Powers

The strength of purpose within your inner powers comes directly from love and truth. These powers do not come from outside you.

You might be wondering how you will ever be able to recognize and use your own inner powers. Take heart because in these pages you will find the most wonderful stories that will resonate with your inner knowing and help bring your own powers to light. Use them to care for yourself, to keep your own healing flame burning brightly.

Your body has infinite intelligence and unceasingly shares all information with you. To heal you only need to look inside and ask yourself, "What do I need?"

Your Inner Power of Protection

Your Inner Power of Protection is an intuitive guidance system working through your emotions. Unflinching in their accuracy, your emotions will always give you correct and truthful information.

To tap into this guidance system, begin to pay attention to how you feel. This is a very simple guidance system with only two measures, one of love and one of fear. Love feels good, fear feels bad. Always go with love in any and all situations. Your Inner Power of Protection will never let you down.

To access your feelings, concentrate on your heart area. Set aside all outside influence for a moment and ask yourself: "Do I want to experience this?" Trust that your heart will give you the right answer.

Today, we have come to realize that environmental factors are having a huge and profound effect on our health. New science shows us that our brain and its thoughts control the genetic expression of our physical body. No longer do we have to believe the dogma that our genes control our life and that we are victims of our 'inherited' weaknesses. We have come to know that the 'gene' theory of disease is completely wrong and that we have immense control of our capacity to heal or to die. (*The Biology of Belief: Unleashing the Power of Consciousness, Matter, & Miracles,* Bruce Lipton, Published by Hay House, 2008)

Fear, toxins, negative thoughts and emotions, unfavorable situations, chemicals, synthetic hormones, a lack of nutrients and an excess of non-nutrients promote 'dis-easing'. Love, sunshine, movement, fresh air, nutritious and appropriate foods, cleansing, rest and relaxation and a positive state of mind enhance healing.

In a recent lecture, author and physician Bruce Lipton shares new discoveries in the science of biology. Consider the nucleus of every cell is the reproductive system, not the brain of the cell. The DNA is not the instruction for how our life plays out; rather it is simply the reproductive system of the cell. It reproduces the cell through replicating its DNA. In humans this determines our physical structure and its expression.

The outer layer of the cell is where all the 'brain' activity happens and where the cell receives signals from the outside world. These signals direct the cell to move either toward growth or away from it. It is the cell's response to the signals that determines whether it follows a pattern of growth and healing or one toward death. If the 'brain' of the cell senses a nutrient, it moves toward that nutrient to engage with it. A cell has thousands of receptors for many different nutrients. If the cell's brain senses a dangerous toxin, it withdraws and moves away. (Lecture 'The New Biology – Where Mind and Matter Meet' by Dr. Bruce Lipton, Retrieved February 21, 2013 from www.youtube.com/watch?v=HVECAlT4AXY)

What does this have to do with healing our body? In our human form, made up of tens of trillions of cells, we also have a brain, which receives signals from nutrients and toxins. In sensing a nutrient such as sunshine, love or nutritious food we will move toward that nutrient, toward growth, reproduction and all the wonderful processes of life. When we sense a toxin, a stressful situation, a negative comment or a nasty chemical, we move away in fear. Sometimes our fear is masked as anger, which is also a good indication that we are trying to avoid something that is in conflict with our best life.

On a chronic and large scale as we face today, we unknowingly allow our poor bodies to be bombarded with negativity throughout every single day. Our standard reaction is one of feelings of fear, anger or despair, which is perpetuated by negative self-talk; constant chatter that feeds and builds on our negative perceptions. Fear and negative self-talk directly suppress our ability to heal. These negative emotions beget poor health. They send energy and blood flow away from our immune system and toward the glands and systems that are designed to deal with the perceived problem, with the stress.

When my mother was in the last few years of her life, she was prescribed Prozac for the depression caused by her poor state of health. I remember how sad I felt after she passed when I acknowledged that she had never been able to express her feelings about what was happening to her, feelings which might have saved her life, had she been able to listen and respond to their meaning.

Your healing system is an inner maestro, always speaking through how you feel. How you feel is the most important indicator of whether you are on the right path toward optimum health. Foster love and healing in your world. Move toward the things that make you feel better, the things that help your body heal. Stop self-sabotage. Love and care for yourself instead.

Your Inner Power of Symptoms

You were blessed at birth with a very powerful healing system, which speaks to you through symptoms.

There are literally thousands of symptoms a person could have. How is it possible to weed through them all to find the answers you need? At first the messages from your body can seem clouded and mixed especially if you are experiencing multiple symptoms.

Symptomatology categorizes symptoms into groups and analyzes their meaning. Groups of symptoms show patterns of disease and this can reveal not only the cause of 'dis-ease,' also what steps should be taken to reverse the damage and overcome illness. Sometimes it can be difficult and take time to work out what your symptoms mean. A symptom analysis can quickly pinpoint which areas need crucial work first in order to effect quick, safe and successful healing.

Certain groups of symptoms are directly related to your body's systems. For example, if you are experiencing discomfort and pain under your right rib cage, along with heartburn and indigestion and an aversion to certain foods (citrus, hot spice, eggs, cooked fats, oils, and rich foods like dairy and meat), it is certain that these symptoms are caused by congestion in the organs of your digestive system, specifically your liver and gall bladder.

You can see how your body is automatically telling you exactly what foods to avoid, to give it a chance to catch up and clean itself out. If you ignore these messages, no doubt you will end up in the operating room, to have your gall bladder surgically removed. This is a last resort, a band-aid designed to deal with the chronic debilitating symptoms of congestion. It's not a step toward removing the congestion in a safe and health promoting way.

Symptoms are your body's way of telling you what is wrong. Ignoring them and covering them up with prescribed medications, alcohol, recreational drugs and addictive behaviors will never help you get to the root of your problem or allow your body to experience life in a way that is beautiful, kind and wondrous. At the worst, ignoring your symptoms can be a fatal mistake.

Your Inner Power of Knowing

The most prominent power that intertwines the stories of people who have cured themselves is that of Inner Knowing. This is an unflinching, stable and Gnostic power, nourished through our experience.

The best example of the Inner Power of Knowing is revealed in Dr. Sue Gelder's story. Dr. Sue was inflicted with a massive tumor at the base of her spine. It was growing blood vessels out from itself, feeding and expanding into her lower body. It brought her to her knees, literally; at one point in her life, Dr. Sue was crawling to the bathroom with one leg atrophied to half its normal size. She was in constant and extreme pain. Doctors said they could do nothing aside from surgery, which would most probably leave her paralyzed, with no assurances that she would be free from the tumor or the excruciating pain. For Dr. Sue, this was not an option. Left to her own devices, at home in bed for eight months, she was able to dissolve the tumor and regain her health completely.

A story of wonder? A miraculous cure? The miracle is that through Dr. Sue's story we are able to recognize it is possible for any one, and all of us to cure whatever 'dis-ease' (challenge) we are presented with. The wonder is that to know and experience your own ability to heal makes your life intensely more beautiful and worth living.

Your Inner Power of Time

Time is something each and every one of us possesses. Time is not gone or wasted. We are not short on time. Time is all we have! The time we have and more importantly, the time we take, is supremely important to healing.

Healing takes time. It is much like tending a garden. It requires trying new things and getting rid of old ones, paying attention to yourself and taking time to assess how you feel. One natural therapy or change in diet won't cure you as much as one medication or conventional treatment won't cure you.

Kapil's story shows best how he used his Inner Power of Time to cure non-Hodgkin's Lymphoma. Kapil's 'dis-ease' began as small pimples on his arms. They spread down his chest, up his neck and onto his face. As the pimples began to fester and become weeping sores Kapil got very sick and began to wonder how much time he had left on this earth.

Kapil didn't give up though and he used the next year to remove his 'train tracks' as he called his toxic mercury fillings, completely cleanse his body and swathe himself in rest and nourishment. Each passing day brought more healing and strength as Kapil's weeping sores began to heal and then disappear. He says that it took only a few weeks before he began to notice a difference. Thankfully he was paying attention. Now more than 20 years later Kapil is happy and healthy and helping others to overcome their own 'dis-eases'.

Take your time to heal. Take your time to rest, to listen and to care for yourself.

Surely it's time for you to experience your own wondrous miracle.

2   Healing Breast Cancer with Divine Intervention

In June of 2008, Linda Devine was diagnosed with breast cancer. At first Linda was deeply disturbed and frightened but with immeasurable courage she stepped away from conventional treatments and chose instead to heal her body naturally, using a simple and healing Macrobiotic diet along with stress reduction and positive lifestyle changes. Here is Linda's incredible story:

I think it is so important for people to know the truth, which is why I am motivated to share my story. In June of 2008, I was diagnosed with breast cancer. I went to a doctor and he found a tiny lump. They decided to do a mammogram, which didn't thrill me, but I agreed. In the mammogram they did see something, so they did an ultrasound and then the doctor confirmed that it was definitely cancer. He recommended surgery and then radiation. I asked him then about natural therapies and he just kind of laughed at me.

I was so scared that I honestly didn't know what to do. I think it was worse because of their attitude. To them it was just routine and not a big deal. I got the feeling that I was just a number, not really a person, you know? Their bedside manner was absolutely horrendous.

The physician made an appointment for me to see an oncologist and immediately scheduled the surgery and radiation. When I left that office, I was in such a stupor that I was just beside myself. The very first thing I thought was: 'Oh my God, I'm going to die, I'm going to die.'

When I really started to think about it though, I thought: 'Its only a little lump. They caught it really early so maybe they can just remove the whole thing and it will be gone.'

I don't believe in the cut and burn thing, that's just not me. Here I was advocating natural health and yet I was considering having this done? Then I kind of got my head back and I decided: 'No, I'm not doing it.'

I talked to them about my choice and they tried to talk me out of it. Basically my doctor fired me.

When I was diagnosed, at that very first appointment, they were already booking surgery and radiation. I was in shock. I didn't have time to even think about it. The doctor told me that if he hadn't been so busy, they would have done it that day. It seems that they don't even want to give you a chance to think. Thank goodness I had that time because my appointment wasn't scheduled for another week.

After the doctor's visit, I knew I couldn't drive home because I was just too shaken up. I walked home instead and in that walk I decided: 'I'm not doing surgery, I'm not doing radiation.' My body just told me: 'No, it's the wrong thing to do.'

It's a horrible situation to find yourself in but once you get past that initial shock, you realize that you are the only person who can take responsibility for your own body, and it's not up to them. You have to find out about what happens to your body and if you really listen to your body, you will know the right thing to do. All the research I did guided me to exactly what I needed to see, what I needed to read and where I needed to go.

I did some research around various diets and foods and what would be the best thing for me, again listening to my body. About six or eight months previous, I'd started doing some research on Macrobiotic eating and it's funny how your body leads you to things like that. I thought there was obviously a reason why I was already led to that, so I did more research on Macrobiotics and it just felt like the right thing, so that's what I did.

I was really, really strict on myself, which is difficult for me because I absolutely love bread; so, no wheat, no gluten, no yeast, nothing like that. That was tough but I did it.

As far as supplements, I took B17, which is Laetrile, for about six months. Every once in a while I think: 'I am okay without it,' and I'm just guided and just listen.

I also took Maitake mushrooms in capsule form, from New Chapters called Host Defense. It's very difficult to get pure Maitake without anything else in it, so there are various other mushrooms in it as well.

I went to a Naturopath who recommended I take Zymactive, which is a proteolytic enzyme. He also suggested I read, *How to Prevent and Treat Cancer with Natural Medicine,* by Dr. Michael Murray. It's an excellent book so I would recommend that too.

I took extra Vitamin C to bowel tolerance, meaning I took a large enough dose to induce diarrhea, then I backed off a slight bit.

I was walking outside quite a bit for Vitamin D so I wasn't taking supplements when I was outside. When I can't get outside as much because of the winter weather, I take a Vitamin D oil supplement. I also take Omega 3, a really good multivitamin, Vitamin A and turmeric.

I did meditation and visualization. In one meditation I actually saw the cells being removed and I just observed instead of trying to control it in any way. I have meditated for years on and off now, every day for five to ten minutes so it's easy to get into that mode of meditation. Even though, there's angst and panic and fear, once you get into that meditative state, that all goes and you can focus on what's in there and what you need to do. You can visualize where the cancer cells are, where the illness is and that's how I guide people, to really just sit with it and be there, be there with whatever it is. Then you can guide your body to do whatever you need it to do.

Regarding nutrition, as I said the macrobiotic diet had shown itself to me so I followed its recommendations, including lots of sea vegetables. Basically the macrobiotic diet is grains, greens and beans; about 40 to 50% grains, about 40 to 50% green vegetables and 10 to 20% beans and other things that you can put into soup.

Miso soup is a big one on the list so I eat it almost every day. The broth is made with fermented organic soybeans and full of beneficial bacteria, which are very important for immunity. Then organic tofu and nourishing strips of Kombu or another sea vegetable are added.

The macrobiotic diet is based on the climate you live in. In our North American climate, leafy greens that point towards the sun are really good for our bodies because we are pulling that energy from the sun. Grains are more nourishing and less troublesome than nightshade vegetables: potatoes, peppers, tomatoes and eggplants. So about half of your intake is whole grains and half vegetables and local fruit and things that grow in this North American climate. That means Swiss chard, kale, spinach, cabbage, apples and carrots. In your climate, it may mean something completely different.

I stopped eating bananas even though they are so rich in potassium. To bring things in that are grown in a completely different climate doesn't gel with our bodies' needs.

The way you cook is also important. Macrobiotics includes lots of chopping and cutting. It considers your frame of mind when you are preparing meals.

It also takes into account the yin and yang energy, which depends on what type of food it is and what kind of energy you need to cure the illness you have.

It's really, really important to stay as positive as you can. This isn't easy because you are scared and you hope you are doing the right thing but you also may have doubts about what you are doing. The key is to use your inner strength to hold that positive state.

Surrounding yourself with positive and supportive people helps as well. If you've got a friend that is rather negative, just remove yourself from that person for a while. Stay away from negative TV shows.

Just focus on yourself, you really need to do that.

I know my cancer is gone because I feel it and I confirmed it with a thermograph exam. In only ten months, I cured my own breast cancer and brought myself back to an excellent state of health and I feel great as well.

I am confident that natural therapies work and I think a lot of people are not quite that confident yet. I know people who believe in natural therapies, then they are diagnosed with a life threatening illness and they let their doctor talk them into conventional treatments. I've seen people die from it. For example, I know a man who developed pancreatic cancer and he agreed to surgery. Afterward it just spread through his whole body.

It doesn't make sense to me, to expose someone to something that is detrimental to their health, when they are already sick. Why would you do that? That doesn't make any sense. It is just heart wrenching when I hear about these things happening to people.

If you have been diagnosed with cancer do research, for your own good, do research.

Stay as positive as you possibly can. I know it's hard, but very important, so stay as positive as you possibly can. Once you pass the initial shock, it gets a little easier and a little easier.

Find a support system. I met some awesome friends who I could talk to, cry on their shoulder and vent to when I needed.

Have faith. Whether you call it God or the Creator or something different, there is a higher power out there, so have faith. It's not meant to be, for you to be sick. Everyone is meant to be healthy but we need to learn to take responsibility for our health. If you just allow others to do it to you, and follow their advice, that's not necessarily the best thing for your body. You have a chance to control your health and your future.

If you are someone who is worried about cancer, and you have not been diagnosed, then meditate and really get into that space and ask: 'Is there anything I should be concerned about, anything that I need to take care of?' You will be guided to the right trail.

Some people believe that macrobiotic cooking is not the right way, because they believe in a raw food diet. That's okay, for some people it's the way to go. The macrobiotic diet is not the answer for everyone but it's certainly healthier than the diet most people are eating and it's providing their body with the nutrients they need. There are many other things out there that are equally as good but this is what suited me.

Taking away all that junk food is the primary problem and what people need to do. Stop going to fast food places. You know you're eating burgers with 'heaven only knows what's in them,' and French-fries, and bags of potato chips. That's garbage for your body. It's horrible stuff. You are filling your body with chemicals and transfigured, damaged fats and depriving your body of the nutrients it needs for protection. That's the main problem.

Adding sea vegetables provides a rich pool of nutrients. There is one dish that I make with Daikon radish. I grate Daikon radish and a whole carrot and boil that with one umeboshi plum, chopped in little pieces. I add small pieces of Nori, the seaweed used to wrap sushi. It's like a soup and it's really good for reducing tumor growth and so many other things.

When you start eating healthy, you will find that healthy foods do so many good things for your body, not just one thing. You have so much more energy and clarity too.

I also used whey protein to help my liver manufacture glutathione, an important antioxidant and cell protector. The macrobiotic diet is a kind of cleanse in itself, but I started on an Isagenix program of shakes with whey protein. The whey protein in their products is not denatured and it hasn't been exposed to any pesticides or any kind of pharmaceuticals. The whey comes from cows in New Zealand, who aren't exposed to pesticides or injected with hormones. It's the purest form of whey protein that you can possibly get and that's what I'm looking for. They also have a product called Ionic Supreme that has about 200 nutrients in it. I took a shot of that every day for a couple of months. Some of these products are expensive but it's your health, and when you are dealing with your health, it's worth it.

Regarding thermograph scanning, it doesn't harm in any way. The more we make people realize what the options are, what is available, that you don't have to do the cut and burn, that its just not necessary; then we all can make intelligent decisions, based on what we know.

There's a lot of information on the Internet, but I would caution people to not take everything seriously that you read on the Internet. Make sure you know what the source is and where it's coming from, because anybody can write anything on the internet, so just be careful where its coming from.

Michio Kushi, Founder of the Kushi Institute, the world's premier macrobiotic education centre, has written several books on macrobiotics and healing, which detail his experience with cancer and nutrition. There are lots of case studies in his books, that outline the treatment given to people with lung cancer — cured;

people with liver cancer — cured; all kinds, skin cancer, and worse, much worse cases than what I've had.

So you know it can be done, absolutely, with no question. I think the most important thing for you to do is to listen to your body and take responsibility for it. That's the biggest thing. It's huge; because there are just too many people that go to their doctor and say I'm sick, fix me. Well, they are normal people just like we are and they don't know what the cure for cancer is.

By Linda Devine

Points To Remember:

- Take responsibility for your body.
- If you really listen to your body, you will know the right thing to do.
- Meditate on a regular basis.
- Use visualization techniques.
- The strict Macrobiotic diet allows 40-50% fresh whole grains, 40-50% green vegetables and 10-20% beans and other allowable foods.
- Take away all junk food and do not go to 'fast-food' restaurants.
- Add sea vegetables for a rich pool of nutrients.
- Eat local whenever possible.
- Stay as positive as you can, do not allow yourself to be scared.
- Surround yourself with supportive people.
- Stay away from negative television and media.
- Have faith.
- Don't allow others to do things to you and blindly follow their advice.
- Take this chance to control your health and future.
- Use thermograph, the safest choice, to screen for breast cancer.
- Don't take everything seriously from the Internet, know who and where the information is coming from.

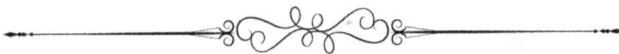

3 Healing Breast and Neck Tumors with a Corrosive Escharotics Paste

When we hear of breast cancer healing stories, we think of strict changes in diet and lifestyle as in the previous story. Although Pattie did use massive diet and lifestyle changes to heal her body permanently, she started with an escharotics paste that burned through her skin and caused her immune system to push four breast tumors and two neck tumors right out of her body. The paste she is talking about in this story is made with a combination of extremely corrosive zinc chloride mixed with water and two powerful cancer-fighting herbs. Greg Caton who invented the paste has been repeatedly threatened by U.S. officials and was incarcerated twice for continuing to market 'Cansema' along with the indication that it cures cancer. Here is Pattie's remarkable story:

Where do I start? As I look back I realized my cancer was a long, hard journey, but the end results; happy, healthy and alive. I did not only cure my cancer, I got rid of irritable bowel, sinus infection, carpel tunnel and a few other ills.

I am not a physician, however, I believe my body was slowly shutting down in 2002. At one point, before I met Greg Caton, I lay on my couch and wanted to die, I was so sick. My grandmother called me from Illinois; she was 101 at that time. She told me to put all of my prescription drugs in the trash, change my diet and so on. Within a week of following her advice, I started to feel better; but I still had to deal with my breast cancer.

My cancer surgeon had scheduled me for breast surgery on a Tuesday in June and I had to confront the fact that I was possibly going to lose my entire breast. I cried a lot. My right breast had a lump the size of a quarter according to the ultrasound and the biopsy was inconclusive for cancer. They wanted to cut on me and had no concrete tests. Despite the emotional roller coaster my doctor had me on, I decided to trust her and go forward with the surgery. I didn't think I had any other choice and was naively allowing doctors to take control of my health.

Then my new life began. A friend of many years, who I hadn't spoken to in over a year called me on the Sunday before my surgery. She had heard from another friend about my upcoming breast surgery. She asked to meet with me immediately and told me to cancel my surgery for the time being.

A few months back I had started a learning session on meditation and regressing into my past lives, what a wonderful trip. The reason I mention this is that I know now, it had everything to do with my cancer journey. I was being led to the right people at the right time to literally save my life.

At this point I was also extremely curious about how my friend healed herself of ovarian cancer without Western medical intervention. I met with my friend at a motel about half way between our houses because of the long distance. She was taking care of her sister at the time, who was taking chemotherapy and needed looking after. Sadly, her sister died in September after doing chemotherapy treatments; she was 51. Her sister trusted her doctors and wanted nothing to do with natural medicine or changing her diet.

She showed me photos of her ovarian cancer tumors, all dead and black, literally falling out of her and I was in awe. I knew and trusted this woman; so I decided to go for it. Besides, what did I have to lose and I thought I might just be able to save my breast. She proceeded to remove the biopsy scab, applied the Cansema and bandaged me up.

It had only been a few hours after applying the Cansema; but, my right breast was so painful, I couldn't go back to sleep. Deb told me it was going to be painful; but this was worse than childbirth. I had no choice but to take a pain pill and then realized I trashed all of my prescriptions. I took the only thing I had left, aspirin. Needless to say, I spent two days in bed, in pain with little sleep. I comforted myself in believing this was better than losing my breasts and it was.

On the third day the sharp pains started to subside and the pain was now a dull, aching pain, which wasn't so bad. Deb told me to take daily photos, which I did. She explained that nobody would believe I ever had cancer if I didn't have proof.

On the tenth day this thing, which was the size of a half dollar, was ready to fall off and I was freaking out. I decided I needed a bath to help relax. I was freaking, because I knew nothing about natural medicines and herbs and thought I might bleed to death when the tumor fell off. I had my cordless phone on the floor in the bathroom just in case I needed to call 911. Looking back, my fear was so unwarranted. The tumor fell off and I decided to save it for more evidence. No bleeding, no pain and I felt absolutely wonderful.

During this ten-day period, I had two pimples on the left side of my neck and they were itching terribly. Deb told me to apply the paste to them and wait and watch. Sure enough, I had cancer somewhere in my neck area. Strange, because I had been going to a specialist for my neck pains and sinus infections for over a year.

What did he do? Nothing but gave me pain pills and steroids. I had also been losing my ability to grasp anything with my left hand and dropped stuff all the time.

I applied the paste and bandaged my neck. This pain was not sharp but dull and not bad at all. The neck tumors, which were the size of a dime, fell off in about ten days. There are a few scars but they are hardly noticeable.

I went to Greg Caton's website and decided to order Cansema tonic and took it for a few months on Greg's recommendation. I was also in contact with Jason Vale at that time because I needed supplement and diet recommendations. I cannot believe I was being led to people who I needed to help me be alive and well.

While my neck tumors were festering, still naive and wanting proof my breast cancer was gone, I made an appointment with my general doctor. She flipped out when she took my neck bandages off and insisted on calling my son for permission to put me in a cancer clinic.

What was her problem? She thought I was a nut I am guessing. I refused to give her my son's phone number and left her office in tears. I did manage to get a few jars of formaldehyde to preserve my breast tumors. I told her I was going to bring them to her for tests, but decided to never go back to her, ever.

Long story shortened, I later went to the county hospital for mammogram and blood tests and didn't tell them anything when asked about my scars. All tests done were negative.

At this point, I am really confused and cannot understand why doctors are not using this for cancer. Thus, my research into natural medicine begins. The first book I read is *Politics in Healing* by Daniel Haley. My awesome angels must be working overtime again.

By Pattie McDonald

Points To Remember:

- Always listen to your grandmother, especially if she is 101 years old.
- Help comes in unusual forms and from unsuspecting people. Always keep an open mind.
- Trust your feelings. If something doesn't feel right, its the best indication that its the wrong path for you.
- Be curious.
- Meditate.
- Take pictures and keep dead tumors for evidence later on.
- Trust that the universe knows what is best for you when it sends you a friend who has already cured herself of ovarian cancer naturally.
- Always have pain medications on hand for emergencies.
- Don't freak out. Stay calm so you can handle situations with intuitive thought and wisdom.
- Seek help from alternative practitioners as well as conventional doctors.
- Look for a skilled alternative practitioner to give you trusted and helpful advice about diet and supplements.
- When you are ready, have tests to be sure you are cancer free.

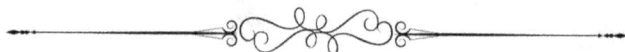

4   Breast Cancer And Cervical Cancer
Annihilated with Holistic Raw Nutrition

Brenda Cobb was diagnosed with not one but two types of cancer, breast and cervical cancer. Brenda's physician told her she would be dead in six months if she refused chemotherapy, radiation and surgery. Brenda didn't buy into the paradigm of 'dis-ease'. Instead, she trusted her own inner guidance and healed herself using an all-natural approach with organic raw and living foods, detoxification, cleansing and emotional healing.

Spurred on by her experiences with cancer, Brenda founded the Living Foods Institute in Atlanta, Georgia and developed her healthy lifestyle program to help people slow and reverse aging and heal all types of disease. Her programs have helped thousands of people from all over the world. Brenda is also a prolific writer and has written many books including the Living Foods Lifestyle. She was awarded an Honorary Cultural Doctorate in Therapeutic Philosophy from the World University and the Pheonix Award by the city of Atlanta as well as numerous awards from other organizations recognizing her amazing work in the field of natural nutrition and healing. Brenda is featured in several movies including 'Healing Cancer from the Inside Out,' and 'The Rave Diet,' which has been used successfully with both cancer and diabetes patients. Brenda is on a mission to teach as many people as possible how to restore and maintain optimum health. Here is Brenda's empowering story:

When I was diagnosed with breast and cervical cancer in 1999, my doctors wanted me to do surgery, chemotherapy and radiation; which many times is the typical mainstream medical approach. I had both family and friends who had been diagnosed with similar cancers and they had done surgery, chemotherapy and radiation and either their treatments had killed them or their cancers had come back with a vengeance. I just knew that going that route would not heal me and I wanted to look for a way that I could heal my body rather than treat the symptoms.

I began my research and on my journey I learned about many people and what they had done naturally. I learned about Dr. Ann Wigmore and her work. I read Eydie Mae Hunsberger's book about healing cancer naturally and that really began my journey. I was so encouraged when I read about other people who had approached health through a natural way. I learned about eating wheat grass juice, energy soup and Rejuvelac and Veggie Kraut. I learned about cleansing my colon and doing wheat grass implants and that was all very foreign to me.

I decided that I was going to release any fear, any negative thoughts that I may have about it and that I was just going to surrender to the process. My feeling was that if others have healed by taking this approach, I could too.

In six months, when my doctor told me that I would be dead, I was not dead. I went back to see him and not only was I alive but all of my cancer was completely gone and he was so amazed that he began sending his patients to my centre.

When I opened the centre it was really starting with the foods. I was thinking it would be just with the foods alone and that would be enough but I learned over time that there were other things that were needed like mental thinking, emotional healing, stress management and reduction and intensive detoxification and cleansing of the body. I learned about adding herbs, essential oils and super foods and so I developed a protocol where people today heal even quicker than I did.

My journey has been one of really healing the body, mind and the spirit so how I got to where I am today really, was listening to my own inner voice. I did a lot of praying and I really felt that I was being guided by God to open a centre and tell as many people about this, to spread the word to let people know that they have options and they have choices and that there is more than one way to look at an issue.

My real inner spirit always told me that in order to heal the body, the natural approach was better. I never resonated with putting a poison like chemotherapy in my body in the name of healing because my good sense told me that poison couldn't be used in the same sentence as healing because if you're poisoning the body, you can't really be healing the body.

I had to change my whole mindset and be willing to do some different things that I had never done before. I had to change my diet. I was born and raised in the South. I had eaten every conceivable animal known to man and of course I ate it the way we love it in the South, fried. I had to change all of that and give up eating all the animals and go to a Vegan diet. Rather than cooking all that food I had to begin to eat it raw and living, sprouted. I was a great gourmet cook before I got involved in this and so that was one of the things that I decided to do. One of my goals was to take delicious cooked food and turn it into gourmet raw and living food. This way everybody would see how delicious it is to get healthy and they would know that they are not deprived.

Nutrition is such an important part of the body's healing process because we need food for energy and fuel for the body. We also need it for rebuilding the body, rebuilding the cells and cleansing the cells. I have found over the thirteen years that I have had my centre, and now have helped many thousands of people from around the world to heal all types of diseases, that nutrition is most definitely important in all of those healing protocols. Our center has programs for Multiple Sclerosis and Parkinson's, Obesity, Schizophrenia, Bipolar disorder, Diabetes, Alzheimer's, Attention Deficit and on and on, pretty much any type of disease you can imagine, even the viral diseases like AIDS, HIV and Hepatitis.

I've learned over time that there are five main, key ingredients to healing and that they actually come in a chronological order of most important. Nutrition even as important as it is actually comes at the bottom of that list. The number one thing that is the most important for people to do to heal is to change their way of thinking because mental thinking is more important than anything, attitude is more important than anything.

The second is emotional healing because there is an emotional component to every disease. Just like people eat for emotional reasons, people also develop diseases based on emotional stuff that sometimes has been buried so deep for so long that they don't even realize consciously that it's there.

The third reason is stress because we know that stress can be a killer. We know that stress can cause heart attacks, it can raise blood pressure, it can cause skin eruptions, heart palpitations. There are so many things that stress can do. So we help our clients to manage stress and learn how to use stress in a positive rather than a negative way. In the world that we live in, we are not going to get rid of stress totally but we certainly can learn how to manage it better.

The number four reason people get sick is that they are full of toxins. They need to work on this by cleansing and detoxifying of the body. We take in so many chemicals, additives, preservatives, colors, and dyes in food and water, through our environment and through the atmosphere. We even take in a lot of toxicity through negative relationships or jobs that we're unhappy in. Toxicity levels can build up and they can really cause serious health issues. We've got to detoxify and cleanse.

The fifth reason, which is the foundation of everything, is nutrition. That's using organic food that is raw, vegetables, nuts, seeds, fruits and sprouted living foods, which are growing when you eat them. Sprouted foods like mung bean sprouts, lentil sprouts, buckwheat sprouts, sunflower sprouts, broccoli and clover sprouts are just some examples. There are a few side things which are very important too like taking in really good, filtered alkaline water, getting fresh air, absorbing sunshine; really to approach holistic balance.

I found that if a person agrees to change what they are eating and even if they decide that they're going to do a pristine organic, raw and living foods diet and they're really good about following it; if they do not have the right mental attitude, if they have emotional stuff that they are not able to heal, if they are stressed out or if they are toxic, the greatest food in the world will not bring them back to perfect health and keep them there. So it really is important, I believe, that everyone understands that it's the synergy of all of this working together.

If you are toxic and you just decide to start eating better food, you're putting good food on top of a toxic situation. If you cleanse your body and you're adding good food, and a lot of foods can assist in cleansing, but if you're cleansing with therapies like colonics, enemas, reflexology, foot bath detox and infrared sauna for example, then your body is able to boost itself up and extract more vitality from the nutrition you're putting in.

I always like to emphasize that we need to look at those five areas together and not just focus only on food.

Many times people will ask me about emotional components for healing and what they should do or how they can really determine what emotional 'stuff,' we'll call it, is creating a particular disease. Normally, I encourage people if they're willing, to schedule a phone consultation with me so I can help them and we can explore more of their individual emotional 'stuff.'

There is always an emotional component. If it's cancer as an example, a lot of times there's grief, anger, repressed feelings that people are holding onto and emotions they are not willing to release from the past. Now cancer can settle in various parts of the body. If it settles in the breast as an example, the emotional component may be that they are over-mothering or over-nurturing to other people, putting everyone else first and putting themselves last, not taking care of their own needs.

If cancer develops in the colon, it can because of a lot of old guilt and old emotions being stuck, with a difficulty in releasing the past.

As I'm exploring these things with the people that I'm working with, most of the time a memory will come up or something will flash for them and I'll ask them: "Does this make sense? Does any of this resonate with you?"

They'll say: "Absolutely, that's just the way I am" or "I remember something that happened in my marriage" or "When I was a young child..."

We can repress those feelings and memories. Women are really good at this because if people say to us: "How are you doing today?" we will say: "Oh, I'm doing great, I'm fine." Maybe we're really not doing fine but we know that most people don't really want to hear the real truth about all the aches and pains we might be experiencing.

When people are experiencing low back pains it usually relates to an emotional feeling of lack of financial support, a fear of not having enough money.

When people have kidney problems, and there are various types and degrees of kidney problems, but a lot of time it's that they literally are 'pissed off' at somebody or even at themselves.

When people have allergies, the first thing I like to ask them is not: "What are you allergic to?" but "Who are you allergic to?" Many times it's about relationships and that we feel kind of allergic to people that we are dealing with and it does take a little bit of time to work with this.

There is a book by Louise Hay called *You Can Heal Your Life* and that has some great information about emotional release. There's another good book called *Feelings Buried Alive Never Die* by Karol K. Truman and that can be helpful. Many times there are forgiveness issues that are wrapped up in this even if we say: "I have forgiven," a lot of times we can be holding on to that un-forgiveness energy when we don't even realize it. There is a book by Colin Tipping called *Radical Forgiveness* and I believe all three of them are excellent readings for anyone who is wanting to begin working on healing their emotional self and really forgiving, releasing and letting go of the past.

If someone has just been diagnosed I believe that it's important if they agree, that we can do a consultation over the phone to look at the whole picture. Not everyone is ready to start at the same place but if someone has a very serious far advanced, lets say like a fourth stage metastasized cancer it really is going to be even more important that they get serious very quickly. A lot of times what I'll do is talk to them and develop a protocol that they can begin at home beginning with diet. Now as an example, even though you may think that fruit would normally be a very healthy thing to eat, it isn't healthy for everybody. In the case of cancer, the fruit sugar can actually be the cancer. In the case of Candida, the overgrowth of yeast in the body, sugar also can feed that. In the case of diabetes, too much sugar and fruit could be detrimental so it's important to have an individualized program.

The protocols I use are not one size fits all and we do like to individualize. If a person is willing to come to Atlanta to my Living Foods Institute, that is the first thing I encourage them to do. If they come right away they can get support, get into the kitchen with us every day and learn how to prepare various recipes. Specifically they will learn which recipes and foods are best for them, they will understand the cleansing and detoxifying therapies, they can work in the emotional healing sessions to heal their emotional stress and they can learn about the various herbs and so forth that are going to support their healing. That way they don't feel alone. When people try to do something like this on their own at home, many times they can get so overwhelmed that they feel like they'll never be able to do it when actually it's a lot easier than what you might think. I think the support and the hands on instruction are most beneficial.

As an example, if you're in the kitchen with us, you're not watching somebody prepare the recipes; you actually get to prepare the recipes yourself. Someone shows you how and then you get to do it and you can imagine how good that makes you feel when you realize: "That's easy, I can do that. I can do that when I go back home."

A few foods that are normally beneficial to everybody are wheatgrass juice and you can start by drinking an ounce of wheatgrass juice a day and build up to three to four or even up to eight ounces, but you have to go slowly with that. We teach people how to also implant wheatgrass in the colon, which can be very healing, very quickly. Scientific research has actually proven that cancer cells, viruses, bacteria and germs cannot live in wheatgrass juice. Wheatgrass can be helpful for cancer and it is also helpful for many other diseases.

There is an energy soup recipe that we use. It's not a cooked soup, but something that is blended in the Vitamix or another high speed blending machine. It includes sprouts, dark green leafy vegetables, a little avocado, a little apple, some sea vegetables and some alkaline water. It's blended into a smoothie or you can blend it thicker and even eat it with a spoon like a soup. It's very cleansing, nourishing, rebuilding and healing.

Then there is a beverage that we teach people to make called Rejuvelac that is fermented and has a lot of friendly bacteria. It not only can help to get the gut, the whole intestinal tract and the colon back into a good balance, it will also help to eliminate the overgrowth of fungus, mold and yeast. Because it's fermented, it also has a lot of extra enzymes and vitamins and minerals in there and it boosts the entire body.

The fourth food that's very powerful for what I call Boot Camp Healing is Veggie Kraut and that is a fermented cabbage kraut, made with cabbage, juniper berries and sea vegetables. It's very easy to make and it keeps for quite a while in the refrigerator. I recommend that everyone eat at least a few tablespoons of that each day, up to half a cup or even a whole cup a day. That can also help in restoring the beneficial bacteria to the colon.

A lot of people don't realize that the colon produces its own B12 with the help of friendly gut bacteria. A lot of people get confused, thinking that the only place they get B12 is from eating meat or animal products but that's not correct. When you have the right amount of friendly bacteria in your colon, you will be producing ample amounts of Vitamin B12.

Points To Remember:

- Make Rejuvelac, which contains pro-biotic bacteria, enzymes, vitamins and proteins and aids in digestion. For a recipe for Rejuvelac by Dr. Ann Wigmore: http://www.youtube.com/watch?v=vs3FaCpHAxE
- Drink Wheatgrass juice.
- Make Energy Soup with sprouts, dark green leafy vegetables, a little avocado, a little apple, some sea vegetables and some alkaline water.
- Make Veggie Kraut with cabbage, juniper berries and sea vegetables.
- Release any fear and negative thoughts and surrender to the healing process.
- Use medicinal herbs.
- Learn about and use healthy oils and fats.
- Total healing includes your mind and spirit as well as your body.
- Listen to your own inner voice.
- Be willing to try new and different things.
- Change your way of thinking and your attitude.
- Practice emotional healing.
- Learn how to manage stress better.
- Do intense cleansing and detoxifying.
- Improve your nutrition by eating nutrient organic, raw vegetables, nuts, seeds, fruits and sprouted living foods.

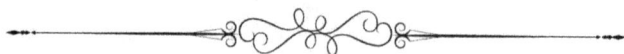

5   Deathly sick with non-Hodgkin's Lymphoma to Vibrant Health

Kapil's illness started many years before he was diagnosed with a very severe case of Non Hodgkin's Lymphoma in 1993. When he finally started to listen to his own intuition and began research that related to his 'dis-ease,' he realized that he had unintentionally caused his own illness. Kapil believes the biggest contributors to his 'dis-ease' were both the extensive mercury fillings in his teeth and his fondness for sweet treats. He immediately eliminated both of these negative toxins from his life and took great steps to trust and follow his own inner guidance. Now in his sixties, Kapil is healthier and happier than ever with no trace of non-Hodgkin's Lymphoma in his body. Here is Kapil's inspiring story:

In 1993 I got hit with a bombshell. I thought I was pretty healthy but I was having these lesions and weeping sores that just wouldn't go away for several years. First I thought it was just a few pimples but then they got bigger and bigger, became open sores and started spreading down my neck and then right down my arms.

I got very concerned so I finally went to a doctor, which I don't like to do very often. I do use the conventional medical system for diagnosis because they are very good at that. Once I know what I am dealing with then I can figure out what to do. I went to the doctor and funny enough he actually queried Lymphoma but the hospital was sending me to the skin clinic and it took them a whole year to finally figure out what it was. When they finally did a biopsy, it was non-Hodgkin's subcutaneous T-Cell Lymphoma. It's a cancer of the lymph system but it primarily manifested on the skin, which in a way I consider very lucky because I could see very quickly when I was having success with what I was doing.

It came as a big shock because I thought I had a fairly healthy lifestyle. For the last forty years I've been into yoga and I meditate twice a day. I was still eating junk food and sweets of course but considerably less than the average person. I have a good mental attitude and so it was a real shock and all my friends couldn't believe it. I thought and they said "Why you?"

It turns out that when I got to the bottom of it, it was caused by massive mercury poisoning from the fillings in my teeth.

It took me a couple days to get over the shock but then straight away I decided: 'No, this is not going to be the end.'

If I managed to create this disease, I can also manage to un-create it.

For anyone looking at dealing with something like that, the first thing I firmly believe that needs to be done is that you take total responsibility for somehow consciously or unconsciously creating what you've got and I think that goes for any disease, any problem.

The doctors told me straight away I needed chemotherapy. I said: "What will that do for me?" They said: "It will give you at least another five years."

I said: "No that's not good enough! It's not enough!"

I hadn't been much interested in cancer before that but when I started looking into it I found the negative aspects of chemotherapy were horrendous. People might live another few years but what sort of quality of life are you going to have? When I researched on the Internet I found that a lot of oncologists would actually not take chemotherapy themselves. That to me says volumes.

I decided straight off that I was going to find a way and it was fortunate timing because I was given the diagnosis one day before the Alternative Medical Fair was starting that weekend in Auckland. I spent a whole weekend going from one alternative healer to the next, over a hundred of them, to find out what I could do and I got over a hundred different answers. I realized there are a lot of solutions out there and a lot of these things are not necessarily suitable for everybody.

I figured the only thing I could do was use my intuition. I gathered all the different ideas that somehow spoke to me. I tried them out and then I stuck with certain things and other things, I decided not to continue.

I was the only one who could decide what was going to work for me and what wasn't going to work for me, and I did this simply by using my intuition, just going by my feelings and what felt right.

One of the healers I went to see was primarily focusing on nutrition and I realized as I learned more and more about it that the nutritional levels are one of the primary things that will affect your immune system. I figured out that my immune system was going to do the healing, so I focused on strengthening my immune system.

I also went for three weeks to a clinic that was focusing on alternative medicine, particularly with cancer cases, to oxygenate my body. I figured out that cancer cells don't grow very well in an oxygen rich environment so I did a lot of oxygenating exercises every day.

When I finally started on my healing journey I was actually very, very, sick by then. It had spread to many parts of my body. My skin was totally grey and I looked half dead already. I had absolutely no energy. The slightest thing would totally exhaust me, so I knew it was really serious and I just had to give it all I had if I wanted to win this one.

It started to improve within a couple of weeks. I was booked in the hospital for checkups every second day and the guys in the white coats put a lot of pressure on me to have chemotherapy. I guess that's how they make their living.

From about the second week on, I saw that it stopped spreading. It was funny because it took about five years before I finally went to the hospital and another year to get diagnosed. The type of cancer I had normally spreads much faster and that's why it took them so long to figure out what it was. I put that down to my healthy lifestyle, particularly I think regular meditation.

By the time they actually diagnosed me it had started spreading quite rapidly. After only two weeks when it stopped spreading, I knew what I was doing was working, so I just kept doing more and more and kept doing the same thing and trying everything that came along.

Intuitively I feel that the work I've done on my nutrition was the most important. I stopped eating any kind of junk food. I love sweet stuff so that was the hardest part. For a year I ate no sugar, no biscuits or sticky buns. That was tough.

One of the very first things I did, was to have all of my teeth with mercury fillings ripped out. I didn't have any money so getting them replaced in a safe way, which is very crucial otherwise you end up with massive mercury poisoning, was very expensive. The government didn't give me any support and I couldn't work anymore because I was far too sick. It was a struggle.

One very kind friend had arranged to have a box of organic fruit and vegetables delivered to my door every week so I tried to only eat organic. I already was very aware of health things, but eating organic was quite expensive. Whenever I could I did and for that year I tried to only eat organic.

I did many different things to detoxify my body because I knew I had to get rid of all that mercury that was poisoning me.

I think it starts in the mind. I totally focused on myself for one year, nothing else was important because if I wasn't going to make it then nothing else mattered.

The other important part was to stop anything that weakened my immune system. The obvious ones are environmental toxins, so I wasn't drinking any more tap water, I was only drinking really high quality pure water because I didn't want all that fluoride and chlorine in my system.

I did workshops dealing with long buried issues about my father, which were gnawing away inside, obviously. Whatever I could come across that sounded promising, I would do it.

Now I'm sixty-five and I have more energy than most kids half my age!

Sometimes when I have a very stressful time in my life, and particularly relationships tend to do that, I will get sort of pimples on my arm again. I would take that as a warning sign and focus again to get rid of whatever the stress was and sometimes that included getting rid of a relationship that was getting too toxic.

Body Balance was developed about twenty-seven years ago and it's a beautiful story, the love of a man for his wife who was dying. The doctors said: "Go home, and make her comfortable, there is nothing we can do," after trying everything they could think of. They didn't know what it was at that stage. Now we know it as Fibromyalgia and Chronic Fatigue.

The man had acquired some knowledge in the past about seaweeds, particularly that the Japanese Okinawa's eat a lot of seaweed. These people have the highest rate of citizens over 100, who are still in very, very good health and enjoying life. They have by far the highest percentage of healthy centenarians in the world.

This man put two-and-two together with divine inspiration from a dream. With the help of a friend who was a nutritionist and scientist, he put Body Balance together. Within just a couple of weeks his wife started improving and within three months she was totally back to normal. Now almost thirty years later, she is a very, very, vibrant, healthy woman. It's a beautiful story.

Body Balance is a live food. It's got every mineral in the planet in it, over 120 different nutrients. It's amazing. Body Balance itself will actually detoxify in an amazing way because the natural ionic minerals will bind themselves to the heavy metal toxic minerals that are stored in the body, that the body can't get rid of on its own, and will chelate them and expel them out of the body.

The important thing is, we never, never promise a cure for anything. This is just food. When the body gets what it needs, it can perform miracles. It's never the therapy that cures cancer; it's always the body, always. It's the body, and we can assist the body to do what it knows to do.

It's my pleasure to share this information and it's become part of my mission in life, my passion, to help as many people as I can and sharing my story sounds like a good way to do it.

By Kapil Arn

Points To Remember:

➢ If you have mercury fillings, have them removed immediately by an experienced professional.

➢ Chelate the remaining mercury from your body using herbs, seaweeds and safe, natural chelating therapies guided by a qualified practitioner if necessary.

➢ Recognize that consciously or unconsciously you have played a part in creating 'dis-ease' in your body.

➢ Do not accept a lesser outcome than that which serves you best.

➢ There are a lot of solutions, each one not necessarily suitable for everyone. Gather the ideas that speak to you, try them all and keep what works best for you.

➢ You are unique and your situation is unique. Decide what will work best for you and what will not work for you by using your intuition. Go by your feelings to determine what feels right for you.

➢ Oxygenate your body at every chance, by exercising outside in the sunshine and fresh air.

➢ Nutrition is ultimately important.

➢ Use nutrition to strengthen your immune system.

➢ Stop eating junk food, all sweets and refined foods.

➢ Eat organic at every chance, every day.

➢ Detoxify your body.

➢ Totally focus on you, nothing else is as important.

➢ Stop doing anything that weakens your immunity.

➢ Avoid environmental toxins.

➢ Drink high quality pure water. Avoid fluoride, chlorine and tap water with additives.

- ➤ Deal with long buried, negative issues that are gnawing away at you.
- ➤ Eat high quality seaweeds or use a supplement made with a variety of seaweeds.
- ➤ When your body gets what it needs it can perform miracles.

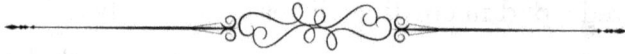

6   A Massive Spinal Tumor Is No Match for a Determined Soul

Left at home to her own devices for almost eight months, Dr. Sue Gelder was able to use the power of her mind through visualization to dissolve the massive tumor that was wrapped around the base of her spine. Now she uses the wisdom she gained through her healing experience to help others heal. No words can describe how amazing this story is except for Dr. Sue's:

I was partway through studying biomedical sciences and I'd been getting backaches and had been going to the chiropractor to try and get it sorted. I wanted to do it myself rather than go to the doctor; I didn't want to go down the medical route.

I had back problems in the past and ended up having an operation, which was successful. This time I thought I would try the natural route but it got worse and worse and the chiropractor actually came out to me to see what was happening. He really didn't know what to do.

The pain was so bad; I literally couldn't even sit up to have a drink. Just going to the bathroom was difficult; it was more than difficult. I had to crawl on my hands and knees just to get to the bathroom and that was literally in the next room.

My doctor came to see me and did give me some medication but really it didn't even do a thing for me. He referred me straight to the hospital but the hospital didn't reply. I was waiting for eight months and just lay in bed with nothing to do. I didn't have a television in my bedroom. I didn't even have a phone in my bedroom so I was just stuck there, wondering what was going on.

The pain radiated all the way down my right leg. What did happen was that I lost half of my right leg, in that it looked half the size, that's the fact of it. It just atrophied completely.

Eventually my daughter came to visit me again, I mean she did that regularly but this particular time I was in so much pain that she rang for the ambulance, which promptly took me to the hospital. They gave me a shot of morphine straight into the vein and that was very welcome. They kept me in for a little while and then they sent me home.

It actually worked for the pain, not completely but it worked temporarily and helped me to rest a little bit because I was having spasms all the way up my spine. The actual pain seemed to be from the bottom of my spine right toward the sacral area, my tailbone.

A few days later I actually ended up going back in the hospital and they kept me in this time. They did the scans and all the MRIs. On this occasion, I think it was the 12th of December 2001, the doctor came to me and he showed the film and said, "You've got a tumor." It was as big as my hand at the base of my spine and it had tentacles coming out and they were wrapping around the nerves coming out of my spinal cord and they were twisting as well. That's why I was in so much pain. That's why every little move was quite painful.

The other thing that he did say was: "I am so, so sorry but I can't do anything. This is not the type of tumor that will respond to chemotherapy. This is not the type that can be radiated away. I don't really want to operate because it will most probably paralyze you and there is no guarantee that you will be out of pain. On top of that, being paralyzed will have additional complications, which could shorten your life very quickly."

Yes they did give me the death sentence. It certainly wasn't long enough. What they do with the kind of tumor that I had was give you three years from the date when they find it. Really nobody expected me to live more than a year and that is in extreme pain. I was on hourly morphine and it really wasn't touching the pain that much either. It really was still very, very painful; so that's where I was.

It was quite interesting that my husband and my friends never talked about it. What did happen was I didn't even tell the family that I had been given the death sentence and I did that deliberately because I knew I would not be able to cope with their grief. I suppose it was being very selfish but at the time that's all I could do. I knew I had to think positive if I was going to get better and I knew I couldn't cope with anything negative. That's how I decided to react to the whole thing.

The fear from the family was only that they never thought I'd be able to get up and walk again. For my own fear, I just decided that this was not going to be the outcome. I wasn't prepared to accept that. I hadn't planned on dying anytime soon anyway and I thought: "How am I going to do this?" That was the big thing.

I think the fear with the doctor was that he could do nothing except give me the medication to help me but really all I had was morphine. That's all I had out of them, just for the pain and it really didn't touch the pain, hardly at all.

What I thought of at that time was how I was going to get out of the pain because it was just stopping me. It was stopping me from healing myself because the pain was so intense. At the time the only thing I knew was that the Chinese are experts at pain management, just by using their mind. That's what I knew, that's all I knew but I didn't know how they did it. I've never read anything about how they did it so I thought I'd just have to figure it out ... and figure it out I did! It took me a few days only.

Apart from the mind, which I mean was absolutely amazing; I actually did visualizations as well, not just thinking about the pain, but how to get rid of the tumor as well. I keep calling it a tumor because that's going to cover a lot of things whether you've got cancer, or non-cancerous tumors, it doesn't matter which. It really makes a difference as to how you deal with it, not what the name of the problem, what the disease or tumor is called.

That's what we come to, is really that diseases, and disease and tumors and cancer or whatever it is that a person's got, really comes from a state of dis-ease, so that the dis-ease becomes disease in natural physical presentation.

Alkalizing the body is absolutely vital. Everybody needs to get to that stage when they've got cancer or any disease, where they really need to look at what they are putting into their body and what is helping their body to repair itself, to renew itself and to change those cancerous or tumor-type cells back into normal cells, or destroy them if necessary.

Food is a big thing as well. Now the fact that I was stuck in bed meant I had definitely changed my diet, in that, I used to like sweets, but I couldn't get out and get them and I wasn't being given them either, so that changed.

There are different types of water that are available. Sometimes the water that comes out of the tap isn't even good enough, especially when you are ill, it's just not good enough. There are different things in my book, *How I Cured My Tumor Naturally and How You May Help Cure Yours Too*, about types of water that are better than tap water to drink and much more accessible to the body even.

It's not about, 'It's my way or no way.' There are certain things that I recommend, some extremely powerful things. If people really want to go down the medical route then by all means that is their choice. I'll tell you what I have found is that when they don't go down the medical route, its a whole lot easier and quicker because then they are not fighting along with medications and things like that. I mean if you're going to go down the medical route, make sure you are very, very healthy in the first place but then you wouldn't be having a problem would you?

The advice I would give to anyone who has just received bad news or a cancer diagnosis is to get a copy of my book, *How I Cured My Tumor Naturally and How You May Help Cure Yours Too*. Yes I'm selling the book and I'm promoting it but there's another reason why I'm saying that. It's because, everything goes out of your mind when you've been given this kind of diagnosis and you just can't think properly at all. If you've got something written down, you'll be able to keep going back to it and back to it and back to it, revising your strategy all the time, rather than trying to figure out what you are going to do and how you are going to work this out. You don't have to go anywhere else, you can just read it time and time again, every day if you have to.

The visualization that I did is very, very specific for tumors of any kind, so it doesn't matter what the tumor is. I would definitely make sure that you get some kind of visualization going, of good health. Try and think being positive and I know that's exceptionally difficult in those circumstances, but you've got to do it.

I think a person really needs to think that just because they've been given the death sentence or some other alternative bad news, it doesn't mean that even though the medical profession can't help anymore or they are extremely challenged with it, doesn't mean that you can't do anything for yourself. I am proof and so are many other people I meet and I've met now since this time. If you decide that you are going to make a difference in your life and you are going to change this outcome, then you most probably will. It's hardly ever the case that you will just die, just like that. It is if you go down the route and you accept the diagnosis, just about everybody dies actually with that diagnosis, if they accept it.

There are things that people can do for themselves, really, really powerful, good things to enhance their life and to make it better. Maybe the tumor will go or the cancer will go completely, I mean I healed and so have my other friends that I've known who have gone down the same route as well as many other people.

Just know that all is not lost ... but that it can be. In my case, I am so, so thankful of that diagnosis and that I was in a place where I couldn't have any treatment. What that did was it made me become responsible for my own health, my own life. I think that's what we need to do, you know? Yes it's very difficult because the mind goes on another journey. It's all about getting the right perspective.

Points To Remember:

> Do not let what others perceive or expect (a 'death' sentence or how long they 'expect' you to live), to become part of your reality. Hold that: '*All things are possible.*'

> Stay positive as much as possible. Do not allow yourself to be affected by negative people and circumstances.

> Be determined to control your outcome. Do not accept anything less.

> You don't need to know 'how' to do something. By being determined about the outcome and asking, 'How do I do this?' as you begin to pay attention the answers will come.

> Visualizations are extremely important to healing, not just thinking about the pain, tumor or 'dis-ease'; visualize dissolving the tumor or illness in a way that is simple and relevant for you.

> It doesn't matter whether you have cancer, a tumor, a cancerous tumor, a non cancerous tumor; what really makes a difference is how you deal with it, not what it is 'called' or how it is 'classified.'

> All kinds of disease, tumors and cancers come from a state of 'dis-ease', which presents itself as physical symptoms and responses.

> Alkalize your body.

> Stop putting harmful things into your body.

> Give your body the things it needs to repair and renew.

> Do not eat sweets and refined carbohydrates.

> Drink high quality alkaline water without Fluoride, Chlorine or additives.

- Write down your strategy and revise it as you go along. This way you will remember why you are doing certain therapies, eating certain foods and you will be motivated to continue those things that serve you and eliminate those things that don't.
- Do the things for yourself, really, really powerful, good things to enhance your life and to make it better.
- Be responsible for your own health, for your own life.
- Hold the right perspective.

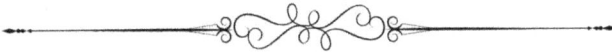

7   Sweet Success for 'Deadly' Black Melanoma

Yvonne was diagnosed with black melanoma and given six weeks to live over thirty years ago. Even though doctors were relentless in their recommendations, Yvonne refused conventional medical intervention and instead traveled to a Mexican cancer clinic to have her tumor removed with a caustic herbal preparation. It took only two weeks before the tumor fell off. Once home back in Australia, Yvonne changed her diet and her exercise regime. She added nutritional supplementation. Most importantly, Yvonne changed her attitudes and thinking around her relationships including her marriage. In short, Yvonne healed her life. Here is her powerful story:

Life gets busy for all of us and it just goes on. One particular day, I noticed that this black mole on my leg was kind of itchy and it changed color and became a bit raised. I thought, 'I don't like the look of that.'

I've never been a person that is sick and I didn't even have a family doctor so I was just at the grocery store and next to the grocery store was a doctor's office, and I thought, 'I'll just pop in there and let him have a look at it because he may ask me to do something.' So I popped in and there was no one else in the waiting room and he came out and he said, 'Yes, he'd like to have a look at my leg,' and the color just drained out of his face when he looked at it. I thought, 'Gosh, poor guy, he's not feeling very well.' He looked at me and started stuttering and then he left me there on the examination table. He went into the next room and started making all these phone calls and he came back into the room and said, "Look, I've got some really good news. I've been able to get you into a specialist tomorrow morning at nine o'clock, so no problems, just go in to the specialist."

So I thought, 'Gosh, what's so serious, so bad.' So the next day I went into the specialist, a skin surgeon in the city and he took me into his room and put me up on the table and took a look at it.

He brought out this gigantic needle and I'm not a needle person so I asked, "What are you going to do?"

He said, "Oh, I'm just going to do a biopsy.

This is how naïve I was, I asked, "What's a biopsy?"

He said, "Well we are just going to cut a bit of this tissue out and send it away to the lab and just check it out."

I thought, 'Oh man, I've got to get out of here.' I was feeling ill in the stomach, looking at this big long needle and I said, "I need to go home, my husband would be so upset if all of me didn't come home." I thought, 'How do I get out of here?'

I ended up talking myself out of it and then I left. I was cold and sweaty and it made me think, 'These guys all think I've got something really wrong with me. These guys want to start slicing me up.'

I went home and my purpose was to contact my Naturopath and ask, "What do I do?"

The Naturopath said, "It would be a good idea to go back and get it checked out because if it is something serious then we can make some decisions about what you can do but if it's nothing, well then you know it's nothing."

I went back that afternoon at five o'clock and the skin surgeon was so cross that I had wasted his time that morning. He stuck this long needle straight into the middle of this black spot, which was about the size of my small fingernail. The pain was so intense that I fainted. They had to resuscitate me and I was in there for about half-an-hour while they were trying to bring me back around.

He said to me, "We'll send it away to the lab and I'll give you a call."

Monday morning he phoned and said, "Good news and bad news. The good news is I want you to come in immediately and we are going to do surgery. The bad news is that it's black melanoma and it's not looking real good; but if you get in here immediately, hopefully we can do something to help you." Then he said, "I hope you haven't been walking on your leg over the weekend."

Well I'd been to a wedding and danced until about three in the morning, which was very interesting. I said to him, "Look I don't want you to do anything, no surgery, nothing. I'm fine."

He said, "You don't understand, this is serious, we need to do something urgently."

I said, "No, no, no. You don't understand. I don't do surgeries."

He said, "Mrs. Chamberlain, if you don't have something done immediately, the maximum we can give you is six weeks to live. The melanoma cells would be released into your bloodstream and we need to look at that leg and probably amputate above the knee joint. We need to do that now. Now. Not tomorrow. Now. Now."

I said, "No, you don't understand. It's not going to happen."

That was my scary impact. I was so scared. I've got three small children. I've never been sick before and he's saying, "You've got six weeks to live."

My husband Ian and I hadn't been getting along really well and I had just told him that I'd had enough of this relationship and that it wasn't working. We didn't talk to each other and we were fighting all the time. I thought, 'Here was a way for me to die and go to heaven and I don't need to let anyone know that our marriage is in a mess.' Then I thought, 'But I don't want to die. What's my option here?'

It was like an avalanche of fear and an avalanche of confusion. It's the insensitiveness of the doctor who just says, "Look you're going to be dead in six weeks." It's the shock too because I'm healthy, I'm well. I'm dancing until three in the morning. 'What do you mean I'm going to die in six weeks?' Die ... dead, you know I was trying to get my head around it.

When I hung up the phone the doctor phoned me back again and said, "Is it because you don't have medical insurance, that you don't want to come in?"

I said, "No you don't understand, I don't do surgeries," and I hung up on him.

Then he rang me back again and he said, "Is it because you're concerned that your leg is going to be amputated? Don't worry about it; we can get you a prosthesis. It's okay."

I guess he realized that he'd come across too heavy so now he was trying to back off, be a bit more gentle and talk me into coming in.

I just said, "No, you don't understand. I'm not coming in. Thank you for your concern. I am not coming in. You've got all of me that you are getting. That's it."

That was early in the morning and I had to wait until my Naturopath opened up so I could ask, "What do I do now?"

The decision was that I would do something alternative and not go for the surgery because I figured if you are going to die in six weeks, why would you die without a leg and go through all that pain and discomfort? My thought was, 'If you die, at least die intact!'

When I went to my naturopath he told me about a clinic that was in Mexico, and he said, "Lets phone them and see what they have to say." We live in Australia and that was the other side of the world. This was early in the morning. I had to wait until the clinic opened and so that waiting time was like mental torture because you start asking yourself, 'Am I doing the right thing? What about my three children?'

People were saying, "You're crazy. People have had surgeries done. It might be okay. Don't procrastinate. This is stupid."

No one had ever heard of an alternate therapy and going to Mexico was considered 'third world.' Why would you want to go to a third world country for cancer treatment?

People said, "Oh, gee, that's terrible. What are your kids going to do?"

It was like an immediate acceptance that you're dead. That's because they believe the medical diagnosis and the medical belief, that I would be dead.

When you have a new belief like alternative healing and no one else around you has done it and you are the first one, it's like being a pioneer. People are scared of that. They think, 'What are you doing?'

I couldn't go down the medical road; that just wasn't my belief structure. The resistance you get from everyone around you, because what you are doing is different, is an incredible challenge.

Ian actually isolated people from me so that they wouldn't infect me with their negative belief structures. Where I'm a very social person, if someone didn't believe that what I was doing was supportive of me and supportive of my goal, Ian just didn't let him or her near me. You are holding on with every ounce of belief you can get and you don't need people cutting away at your thin thread of belief. It was just an isolation tactic really.

I ended up going to Mexico even though I didn't have a passport, I didn't have a visa. This was Monday. I had spiritual faith and I just said, 'Well God, you know that I need a visa and a passport because I can't get there without it and I haven't got a lot of time to get that.' You ask for guidance and guidance will come, if you're open to it. A thought popped into my head about a person I had met years earlier that was now an Australian Senator, so I phoned him up and I said, "I need to get a visa and a passport to the U.S." I told him why and he said, "Well here, use my name, here's how you do it."

I had the documents in two days and I was on the plane on Wednesday morning. It was just a miracle because normally visas and passports take three or four weeks. It was one miracle after another.

I was in Mexico for about two weeks and the reason why was because it was an external cancer so they needed to do a longer treatment. Where as if you go to that clinic, and there's stacks of clinics in Mexico, and depending on what kind of cancer you have, that determines how long you need to be there. Some clinics hospitalize you because of the treatment. For some people it's an outpatient situation. I was actually there for two weeks and they treated the cancer externally. I saw it drying every single day. In front of your eyes, you just see this thing withering up. It was amazing!

I could see what was happening on my leg externally but then I still had that element of doubt, 'What if it doesn't work?' I started doing research on what else I needed to do.

I got a hold of some books to help me in my thinking. There was a book written by Dr. Maxwell Maltz called Psycho-Cybernetics. It's a pretty heavy book to read but I read this book and it explained the power of your mind to heal your body. I started realizing that I had to believe what I was doing was the right thing. Then I came to understand the power of your mind and negative thoughts and how destructive they could be. I started examining what had brought me to that point in my life and realized that my mental thought process, my negativity, my anger, my resentment, my bitterness, my wanting to get even; this huge plethora of negative, angry emotions had brought me to this point in my life where I was not liking me and not liking the world that I was in. Then your mind goes into the solution and says, 'Well if you don't like you and you don't like the world that you're in, I'll take you out of it because that's what you are telling me, so consciously that is what you want.'

That reality, that realization was such a shock to my system that I began just reading everything I could get my hands on about the way the mind controls the outcome in our lives and it was just an ugly realization for me, but a true realization.

The first thing that happened to me was the revelation that we can change our thoughts. I didn't think that we could because thoughts just happen; a thought is something that just comes into your mind. I wondered how do I take control of these negative thoughts? I realized that some of those negative thoughts came from my negative attitude, so by changing my attitudes I would then change the thoughts. So the attitude was a belief structure that I had embedded in my psyche from previous programming from my parents, from teachers, from peer groups, from media. You have these attitudes and belief structures.

I realized that I had taken on board everything that has been said to me. I recognized that I needed to make my own decisions about what I believed and as I started evaluating my value systems and my belief structures I was able to ask, 'Where did that thought and belief come from?'

I was able to then choose whether I wanted to keep that belief and ask is it serving me or is it not serving me? I was able to then decide when a negative thought would come in, to evaluate it, and ask, 'Where did that thought come from?'

Sometimes it worked to replace that negative thought with a positive thought.

If I say to you, "Don't think about pink elephants." Straight away you think about pink elephants.

You can't say, don't think about something because the moment you say don't think about it, you think about it! The only way to get rid of a negative thought like, 'You're going to die' was to change that negative thought to a positive affirmation and say, 'I choose to live, I choose to live!'

When a negative thought would come in, I changed it to a positive thought or maybe even challenged the thought and said, "That's what the doctors think but that isn't what I've chosen." That was another way that I changed it. I used a variety of ways to try and control the brain cells that never in the past had been controlled at all.

Awareness is the first key, to identify that I am thinking that thought first of all. I was never aware of my thoughts before, they were just in my head. Thoughts of 'poor me,' 'this is not fair,' just victim mentality and victim mentality is a thought process. I didn't realize that I was indulging in the party of 'poor little old me' and inviting other people to join me.

I'd go to the hairdresser and make a negative comment about my husband and what had happened and everyone would join in and it was bigger and better and more horrible and more vicious. You're just feeding that negative belief structure that men are awful. Well who said? You can choose to see all the negative in your partner or you can choose to see all the good.

I had to realize that I was focusing on the negative and people around me were reinforcing that by saying, "Well yeah, my husband does that too, yeah my neighbor, yeah my dad, yeah my brothers." It was just constantly reinforcing that belief and making it stronger and stronger. I had to identify with what I was doing, and say, "I created that belief brick by brick and now I have to take it down brick by brick." I did it by saying, "This was the good stuff that I saw in him when we fell in love." When you start focusing on the good instead of the bad, your whole attitude toward a person, toward a situation, toward a circumstance starts to change. The changes that happened in our relationship when I started to see the good instead of the bad were just remarkable.

My life was a gift. When my mother gave birth to me, it was a gift. What I do with my life is up to me. When we are trying to please everybody else and doing what everybody else thinks we should do, the 'shoulds' can get us down. When you are not doing what you *should* do, you can feel guilty then you feel as though you have to blame or justify things. One of the things I did was just get rid of the '*should's.*' We have a joke now and we say, "Have you been *should* on lately?"

I chose to get that word out of my life and out of my diary, out of my dictionary. Instead of saying should, I say could, I could do this and by saying I could, it gives me the power of choice. When you have the power of choice it means you are responsible and you are also accountable. That just changed me. I had to ask myself if I would take personal responsibility for the actions that I was doing in my life because up until that point in my life it was his fault, her fault, my mom's fault, my dad's fault, it was everybody else's fault, not mine.

If you get rid of the '*shoulds*', you can get rid of blame, you can get rid of guilt, you can get rid of fault. That just gets rid of so many negative feelings, just by saying, 'I could' instead of 'I should.'

Our words have energy so I started evaluating the word that I was saying and asked, 'What energy is behind that word?'

Our words come from our heart, our belief structure and our value system so it's important to understand the energy that those words have and what those words will do.

Think of something simple like saying, "My cancer." My is a possessive pronoun and if I am trying to get rid of something, why do I keep claiming it by saying, "My cancer?"

I had to realize I was claiming the cancer when I said, "My cancer." We care for and protect our belongings and I had to realize I was possessing the cancer when I said, "My cancer." Instead of saying, "My cancer" I changed that one word, "My" to "This." This cancer, not my cancer because this cancer, this, is something that you can discard but if it's mine, I own it and there is great power in those words. Everybody talks about, "My cancer." You hear it all the time and then they are trying to get rid of something they are claiming as their own.

Cancer is not final. Cancer is a stepping-stone to identifying your true purpose and your true destiny.

It's my pleasure and a total joy to share my story. Hopefully people can take something to support them on their journey.

I'm motivated to bring out my story because somebody helped me and it's not just about me, it's about all of us together. We are on a journey against a disease called cancer. That's all it is, it's a disease and diseases can be conquered.

It's kind of like that movie, 'Play It Forward'. You can't receive and be greedy and hold onto it; it's about giving it out. There have been other people who have decided to go natural from my recommendation combined with their own research. I have been another link to give them faith and belief to hold on to.

You can change your physical body. You can do it and all you need to know is that other people have done it. That gives you the belief, 'Possible in the world, possible for me.'

If I can do what they've done then it can work for you as well. That's it. I can't have had this amazing miracle for myself and not share it with people. Other people have purpose and a destiny as well and if I can make a difference, that to me is my total satisfaction.

By Yvonne Chamberlain

Points To Remember:

- Trust yourself.
- Do not allow others to instill fear or panic in you.
- Consult with a qualified natural practitioner for support and guidance.
- Educate your friends and loved ones so they do not experience fear around your 'dis-ease.' Ensure them that you are making the right decision for yourself.
- Do not let the opinions of others, who may not be as informed as you, affect your decisions or make you feel guilty about your choices.
- If people are not supportive of you or your goal, stay away and find people who are supportive.
- Have an open mind.
- It's important to believe that what you are doing is the right thing. If you feel conflict inside, then you must take the time to reassess and adjust your path.
- Examine what has brought you to this point in your life. Is your mental thought and attitude having a negative effect on your health?
- Be aware first. Whenever a negative thought enters your mind ask, "Where did this negative thought or belief come from?"
- Adjust your belief structure and replace the negative. For example, a negative thought like, 'I'm going to die' can be translated to a positive affirmation like, 'I choose to live, I choose to live!'
- Do not engage in negative conversation.
- Your life is a gift. What you do with your life is up to you.

- ➢ Get rid of the 'shoulds.'
- ➢ Understand the words you think and speak have either positive or negative energies attached to them.
- ➢ Do not claim and possess your cancer by calling it 'My cancer.'
- ➢ Cancer is not final. It can be used as a stepping-stone to identify your true purpose and your true destiny.
- ➢ Diseases can be conquered.
- ➢ Possible in the world means possible for you.

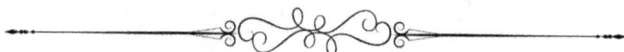

8 Colon Cancer Conquest with Surgery and Raw Nutrition

At only 26 years of age Chris Wark was hit with the devastating news that he, self-proclaimed 'Barbecue King', had Stage 3 Colon Cancer. After doctors removed the tumor in Chris's colon he had a difficult decision to make about what treatments to go with. Chemotherapy would most probably make him sterile and he and his wife were planning on having children in the very near future. Chris had only one choice. Guided by unshakeable faith, Chris used a 'man-style' and very simple version of the raw food diet to kill any remaining cancer in his body. Here is Chris's liberating story:

I was diagnosed with Stage 3 colon cancer when I was 26 years old. After surgery, the oncologist told me I needed to do six to nine months of chemotherapy. I did not have a good feeling about that. My wife and I actually prayed that if there were another way besides chemotherapy that God would just open the door. Two days later I got a book on my doorstep called *God's Way To Ultimate Health,* written by George Malkmus. He had colon cancer about thirty years ago and beat it with nutrition and natural therapies. He did not have surgery or chemotherapy. As I was reading that book I knew it was an answer to prayer and I thought, 'This is clearly what I need to be doing.'

We met with the oncologist and we asked him if there were any alternative therapies available. He said, "No, there are none."

I asked him about the raw vegan diet. He said, "You can't do the raw vegan diet, it will fight the chemo." He told me if I didn't do chemotherapy that I was insane.

We went home and adopted the Raw Vegan diet. I did that for 90 days straight with juice fasting and only raw fruits and vegetables and seeds and nuts. I ate no meat, no dairy and no processed food. After that I was working with a Naturopath and he put me back on a diet with some clean meat, more of a Paleo diet. I ate lots of raw fruits and vegetables, about 80% raw and the other 20% was clean organic meats and a little bit of complex starches and grains like sweet potato, organic brown rice and quinoa. I stuck with that diet along with a lot of natural therapies and herbal supplements for several years and had my blood tested every month. I did CAT-Scans and the cancer never came back. I'm now 35 years old.

The medical establishment, especially oncology, uses fear to manipulate patients into jumping on the conveyor belt and following the doctor's prescription, which usually includes getting on pharmaceuticals, doing surgery, taking radiation and chemotherapy. These are very, very destructive therapies.

I had surgery and I'm not completely against surgery. In some cases I think it can help give your body a jump-start toward fighting cancer.

They use the fear of dying to motivate you to take action immediately. I believe any decision that is a fear-based decision is a bad one. The best decisions are faith based, not fear based.

They told me, "Look if you don't do this, you're going to die."

Often, people go along with it and say, "Okay, just tell me what to do."

I knew deep down that was not the path for me. My kids are young. I have two girls and they're three and six years old. If I had agreed to chemotherapy, I would probably be sterile. That was another reason why I didn't want to do it because I had plans to live. I thought, 'Yes, I've got this cancer diagnosis but I'm going to live, I'm going to beat it. I'm going to transform my health, I'm going to radically change my diet and lifestyle, take control of my health and make plans for the future. That plan included having a family.

To me, chemotherapy didn't make sense because first, it's so destructive it destroys your immune system and your immune system is what keeps you well. Even if you have cancer, your immune system is still working. It may not be working at its peak efficiency, it may be suppressed, your body may be overloaded with toxins, or both, but destroying the immune system can cause any cancer cells remaining in your body to just explode after the chemotherapy treatments. I see it over and over again. People that do chemotherapy always seem to have the same story. They do the chemotherapy and the cancer is gone for a short term. In most cases it comes back with a vengeance, it takes over his or her entire body and everybody wonders what happened. It's very clear what happened. Their immune system was destroyed. Chemotherapy is highly toxic, its a carcinogen, it causes secondary cancers, plus it makes you sterile.

I was looking at all these negatives and then the doctors told me that if I did chemotherapy, I had a 60% chance of living only five years. When I added all that up, it didn't sound like a great option, and I thought, 'I'm going to look elsewhere.'

A lot of people don't understand this until they are in the cancer situation but there's a lot of emotional and social pressure to do chemotherapy; to follow your doctor's orders, to not question anything they tell you and just to say, "Yes" and take it. That was the most difficult part. I had well meaning family members that love me and care about me who were telling me I was crazy and I was making a mistake and I was dying and I had to do what the doctor said.

The other component was the faith aspect. I prayed that God would lead me in the path of healing. Along the way he constantly reminded me that what I was doing, was the right thing and he put people in my life and signs and signposts along the way. That helped a lot.

If you have cancer and you're reading this and you're trying to decide what to do, whether to pursue nutrition and natural therapies or to pursue conventional therapies, be prepared for some opposition. Be prepared for some ugly conversations with your doctors. Be prepared for people who will tell you, "You're crazy and you're a fool." If you're prepared maybe it won't sting as bad when it happens.

Chemotherapy is so destructive. The oncologist told me I couldn't do the raw food diet and chemotherapy together because the raw food diet is a very aggressive detoxification and healing diet. When you convert from a diet of processed foods and animal products and the 'Standard American Diet', to a raw fruits and vegetables diet, with a lot of vegetable juice and periods of juice fasting, your body just starts to detoxify rapidly. It starts burning through fat and you go into 'ketosis', which is burning through fat for energy.

Your body stores toxins inside fat cells so toxins that are stored up are being released for elimination and your body kicks into housecleaning mode. Especially when you fast, your body has excess energy that it can use to repair itself, that would normally be used to digest food. When you are not eating, your body uses that energy to repair itself.

Chemotherapy and raw nutrition don't work together because when you're eating raw foods it will kick the chemotherapy out very rapidly and the chemotherapy won't work. That's why doctors tell you that you can't do chemotherapy and a raw food diet at the same time.

Because chemotherapy destroys your immune system, you are more susceptible to bacterial infections and all kinds of problems just from eating a raw piece of fruit. If there is any bacteria on a raw piece of fruit, normally it's not a problem for you but when you're immune system is decimated, that bacteria can become a real problem.

People ask me all the time, "Can I do alternative therapies with chemotherapy?" You really can't. There is very little benefit because when you are on chemotherapy, doctors will tell you that you have to eat cooked food. They literally tell you, go home and drink a milkshake; we want to keep your weight up. You can't be eating junk food like ice cream and milkshakes just to keep your calories up to maintain your body weight. This is very counter-productive to healing.

My strategy was to overdose on nutrition so I was putting more raw nutrients into my body than it needed. I added an overabundance of nutrients through supplements, juicing, raw foods and raw fruits and vegetables. I intuitively believe that my body is designed to heal itself and if given the proper nutrients that it *will* heal itself.

I came to the realization that the way I'd been eating and the way I had been living was starving my body of nutrients. I was eating a lot and getting full but I was eating dead food. I was eating fast food every day. I was eating microwave dinners, drinking sodas and eating candy bars. I've always been thin and never worried about my weight. I thought I had a free pass and I made really bad decisions about my diet. I was like the 'Junk Food King.' I was a barbecue connoisseur. I love barbeque. Don't eat it now.

Once I realized that I was starving my body of nutrients, then I thought, 'Okay, maybe I can take responsibility for that. Maybe I'm contributing to my sickness and if so, then I can contribute to my health.' I think that's a big lesson that a lot of people need to learn. We have been ingrained to think that if you're sick it has nothing to do with you at all, that it's just a random coincidence, something that's happened to you. You're a victim if you're sick and the doctor has the cure for your illness, which is a patented prescription pharmaceutical drug. There is nothing in nature that can help you. Only patented pharmaceutical drugs can help you.' Right? That's the mindset that we've been conditioned to believe and I grew up believing that too. However, I've always been a little suspicious, especially about pharmaceutical drugs in general.

I made a choice to overdose on nutrition. I believe that our bodies are intelligently designed to heal, that the earth was designed to support human life and that on the earth are fruits, vegetables, seeds, nuts and herbs that all contain vital nutrients that our body can use to heal itself.

I'm still here, eight years later. There's no guarantee that I'll live forever, right? I'm going to die at some point. I don't know how I'm going to die but I've beaten the odds. For eight years, I've beaten the odds. I don't have cancer today so I'm super happy with the choice I made.

My opinion is that if you're sick you should first radically change your diet and lifestyle. Examine every area of your life that may be contributing to your disease and there are probably things in your life that are contributing to your sickness that you don't realize. If I knew then what I know now, I might not have had surgery. I was rushed into surgery right away, which is standard. As soon as you get the diagnosis, they act like there's not a minute to spare, that you've got to have surgery immediately and everything is just rush, rush.

If you're diagnosed with cancer and the doctor says that you need to have surgery in thirty days, then radically change your diet and lifestyle right now. Go to a strict, raw vegan diet, raw fruits and vegetables, giant salads, fruit smoothies, lots of carrot juice and vegetable juice. Avoid fruit juice because it's too sweet but fruit smoothies are okay. Do that for thirty days, up until a few days before your surgery. Go back to the doctor and have him look at your blood work. Have him do some tests and see if you haven't made any progress. Chances are when you make that kind of radical shift, everybody is different and some people heal faster than others, but there's a good chance that they're going to look at your blood work and your scans and see an improvement. If they see an improvement that means you're on the right track and you have a justifiable reason to say, "Hey listen, I want to keep doing what I'm doing, I think this is working. I'd like to push the surgery off another two weeks or another four weeks and keep doing what I'm doing, because I feel like I'm getting better and even your tests show I'm getting better." I think that's a very doable strategy for anyone with cancer.

Now occasionally there will be a situation where a person has to have surgery because their life is at stake, for example, there's a tumor that's blocking their windpipe.

If you are in a situation where you have some time, and the doctors say, "Yes, look you do have a few weeks" or "Yes you could take a month," you could say, "I think I'm just not taking care of myself. I really want to just completely transform my health and see what happens."

They'll probably tell you, "Oh its not going to help," but that doesn't matter, you can still do it anyway. It's your choice.

No one is going to take better care of you as a patient than you will, if you decide to treat yourself.

That's my best encouraging advice to people. Take a radical, massive, action plan and put it together. I detail everything on my site and here it is in short:

My Step 1

I drank eight servings of vegetable juice every day, eight-ounce servings. I bought a Champion juicer. I juiced enough juice in the morning to last me throughout the day and I stored it in little airtight mason jars.

My Step 2

I ate giant salads for lunch and dinner. I'm talking about every vegetable you can cram in a huge bowl. I ate cauliflower, broccoli, kale, spinach, onions, red, green and yellow peppers, mushrooms, sprouts, and nuts. I just crammed it all in there and made a homemade salad dressing with olive oil and Apple Cider Vinegar. Just an oil and vinegar dressing, it's delicious and anybody can do that. Then I would top it with four cancer-fighting spices: garlic powder, oregano leaves, cayenne pepper and powdered turmeric root. I ate that giant salad every day for lunch and dinner.

My Step 3

I made a fruit smoothie in the afternoon with a young coconut. I pour out the juice and scoop out the meat and put it all in a blender. Blend it with two cups of frozen organic berries and that can be a mixture of blueberries, blackberries, raspberries and strawberries. Add a banana if you want. It's delicious and very high in antioxidants.

Coconuts have this amazing medium chain fatty acid called Lauric Acid, which is super, super good for you and it also has calories so it helps maintain your weight. The raw vegan diet is a very low calorie diet. Fruits and vegetables don't have very many calories. They are nutrient dense but they are very low in calories.

That was it. I did that for ninety days and there were periods where I would do a strict juice fast for maybe three to seven days. I didn't follow a very specific schedule, I just did it several times during that period and then I did it several more times in the next couple of years. That was my basic meal strategy and I did the same thing every day. My point is to keep it simple. Just give me something that works. I want to get the most nutrients in my body as I can, every day and I don't want to think about it, so that was my really simple plan.

On top of that I took a lot of different supplements that were prescribed by my Naturopath and other things I had read about. I read a ton of books.

The diet is foundational and supplements are supplemental and I think people get confused and they think well, 'I have cancer and I'm going to do chemotherapy but I'm also going to drink this tea.' Then the cancer comes back and all of a sudden they say, "Oh alternative therapies don't work because I tried one, I tried this tea and I still have cancer." Do you know what I mean?

What I recommend to anyone is if you're going to do it, go all the way, hard-core diet change. Start exercising, walk, run or do light cardio because you've got to sweat to get the toxins out of your body, sweating is so important. Do that *on top of* the supplements that you read about that might boost your immune system or help you detoxify.

I'm one of many and the thing is the world doesn't know that I'm one of many. They think I'm an anomaly. You get this reaction sometimes, "He was just lucky or it was a fluke, or that's anecdotal." You know you can go by, "Just because he didn't do chemotherapy doesn't mean you shouldn't." There are thousands and thousands of people who have done what I've done. They've used nutrition and natural therapies to heal themselves from every kind of disease.

Diet was such a big thing for me; Hippocrates said it best, "Let Food Be Thy Medicine and Medicine Be Thy Food."

How can a person heal? With Food, Faith and Fun!

By Chris Wark

Points To Remember:

➢ Do not allow others to instill fear in you.

➢ Do not buy into the 'fear of dying.'

➢ The worst decisions are fear based. The best decisions are faith based.

➢ Trust your inner instincts.

➢ Decide to radically change your diet and lifestyle. Transform your health. Take control of your health. Make plans for the future.

➢ Do not do things that suppress your immune system's vital functions.

➢ Weigh the negatives and positives and make informed decisions, ones that are logical and make sense to you.

➢ Don't just follow along with someone else's agenda and do what you are told.

➢ Be prepared for resistance from well meaning friends and family members if you decide not to follow the status quo.

➢ Have faith. Be open to guiding signs from people, books, research and other messengers.

➢ When you fast your body uses excess energy to clean and repair itself.

- Chemotherapy and raw nutrition don't work together. Super nutrition kicks the chemotherapy out very rapidly and it won't work.
- Overdose on nutrition and keep it simple.
- Your body is designed to heal itself when given the proper nutrients.
- My protocol Step 1: Eight, eight-ounce servings of fresh-juiced vegetables every day. Step 2: A giant salad for lunch and dinner with four cancer fighting spices: garlic powder, oregano leaves, cayenne pepper and powdered turmeric root. Step 3: Fruit smoothie with one young coconut, two cups of organic berries.
- Coconuts have medium chain fatty acid Lauric Acid that helps to maintain your weight.
- Heal with Food, Faith and Fun!

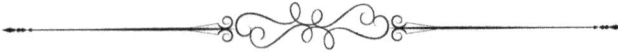

9   Healing non-Hodgkin's Lymphoma
Packaged In Love And Care

With the past experience of watching her mother die from uterine cancer and chemotherapy treatments, Nuro knew that toxic chemotherapy and radioactive treatments did not sit right with her. Instead of being pressured into something that Nuro felt wasn't for her, she chose to follow and trust her inner voice. Though doctors said Nuro would become 'very weak,' her natural path created unwavering strength. Instead she became physically and spiritually stronger with every passing day as her focus shifted away from being sick and toward becoming stronger. Here is Nuro's beautiful story:

In 2009 I was diagnosed with non-Hodgkin's Lymphoma, Stage 1 and I was told it was an aggressive one. I was advised to have chemotherapy straight away. Prior to this I had found a little lump in my breast. In the U.K. the health system is very quick to send women to breast screening if they suspect breast cancer. That in a way was my luck. After several investigations and tests I was told that I don't have breast cancer, what was assumed, but that I had Lymphoma, a type of lymphatic cancer in a very unusual place. It wasn't in my lymph nodes; it was just in my breast a bit away from my lymph nodes.

I was really shocked like anybody would be, because I considered myself fairly healthy. I don't particularly drink in excess. I'm a Massage Therapist so bodies constantly surround me and I can see what a healthy body is and what an unhealthy body is. Nevertheless, here I was with non-Hodgkin's Lymphoma. I was sent to the lymphoma clinic and I was told after several tests that it is an aggressive type. That means it's fast spreading. I was told that I should start with chemotherapy straight away, which would be most probably followed by radiotherapy. I thought, 'Whoa, wait a minute.' I had seen my mom dying from cancer of the uterus. She was one of those patients who did everything that the doctor wanted her to do. She had a dreadful ending.

I heard about a friend that had cured herself of cancer for the second time, once when she was a child and her parents had put her on the Gerson Therapy and now some forty years later she again had a cancer diagnosis and cured herself with natural medicine. That really got my light bulbs going and I thought, 'There must be something else.' In total desperation and total shock I rang her up and said, "What can I do?"

She sent me a whole list, an emergency list of what I could do. She said stay away from all food that is acid forming and go onto a very clean diet. She sent me lots of things but the only things I remembered were that I needed to have a very clean diet and I didn't want to make any decisions out of fear. Obviously I was gripped by fear and panic and had these doctors in my ear and on my case, wanting me to start chemotherapy the following week. So I went on this very clean, mostly vegetable diet, with lots of fresh green juices. I thought, 'I need to buy time. I need to find a sympathetic doctor who likes that I tried to cure cancer without chemotherapy.'

That was all I could think of. I couldn't really research or get further down into this whole thing because I was just terrified. Meanwhile my husband was on the computer and looking at all kinds of possibilities of what I should be doing. After about three weeks I got my head around and I thought, 'Right, I really need to take this on. I really need to regain my strength and my power. I'm not just this victim that's laying down to die.'

I got this letter saying, "Ms. Weidemann has this irrational fear of chemotherapy and we think if she doesn't go down this route she will be dead within six months to two years." So that's three and a half years ago, I'm still alive and kicking.

I learned more and more about how to cleanse my body through food and also I practice a lot of naturopathic methods. I realized a lot of people do a similar routine and it meant that every day I did a coffee enema and a castor oil pack over my liver. I did meditations and I stopped working for several months. I lay out in the sun to absorb Vitamin D; in moderation obviously not for hours, it was a short time.

More and more my body just felt so strong and it wasn't just my body, I felt my spirit really was with me all the way. I mean if you think of a cancer patient you think of this person who is really down in the dumps and very ill. It might sound strange, for me it was one of the best months of my life. It was like I had this little private spa at home and it was a beautiful summer and I just took care of myself for months. I just thought, 'What is it that makes me happy? Eating healthy food makes me happy. Doing alternative treatments makes me happy.' Some people asked, "Oh isn't it exhausting? Isn't it boring?" For me it was fascinating how my body kicked in to embrace all these things. I discovered my creativity again. I started a pottery course, which I'm still doing. I felt stronger and stronger.

In between I wanted to keep up the connections with the doctors here. I wanted to stay in the system because they are very good at giving you a diagnosis. Their treatment, I don't agree with. I wanted to know what I was dealing with so I went there.

It was very obvious that even though I had a lumpectomy on my breast where they had taken the initial lump out, a lump actually had grown back much bigger than the lump that was originally there. In a way that's almost textbook. Naturopathy teaches the tumor is the tip of the iceberg. The cancer was in the whole system and the tumor was a manifestation of the cancer.

I went there every other month and they measured the tumor and the tumor basically stayed the same, always about two to three centimeters. It was obvious too. I had this little bulb on my breast but I wasn't too concerned because in my general spirit I felt good.

I went back to the doctor and I said, "Maybe you made a mistake because I feel good. Yes I have this lump but I feel good."

They said, "Look we also saw that we might have made a mistake. We checked your tissue sample. It's very obvious that it is non-Hodgkin's Lymphoma."

I asked, "Yes but what can I do if this spreads? I don't really have any major symptoms so how can I know if it spreads to other parts that aren't obvious to me?"

They kept on saying, "You will feel very weak."

I kept on checking and I didn't feel very weak. I went walking every day. We live right by the sea on the English Channel, near the cliffs. There is one walk to the beach where I had to go up and down a huge staircase every day. I thought, 'Okay if I don't manage the staircase anymore I have to go into another gear,' but I kept on trekking. I felt stronger and stronger. After about a year and a half, I started to work slowly again giving massage sessions, but only bit-by-bit, I really took it on my own terms.

I went back to the doctor and they performed one test that was quite crucial. I said, "I want to have this test again because I think my cancer is gone," because this lump on my breast eventually became very hard and then it just disappeared. I think it broke up and was reabsorbed by my body and eliminated. Even though he said, "Oh I don't know if it is actually the time yet," he did the test and the test came back that there was no cancer to be found.

The general belief is that you can only cure cancer by chemotherapy, radiotherapy and surgery. In England, any doctor who says that healing cancer is possible in a different way is basically stepping outside of his boundaries. They are not allowed to say this. When you are first diagnosed with cancer there is so much fear coming up. Members of the medical profession present them selves with such confidence. For example, I was told that the type of cancer I had has a very good chance of being cured with chemotherapy. Now that might well be the case and in my eyes, chemotherapy in itself is such an aggressive form of treatment that you might get rid of the cancer and you might develop loads of other diseases or illnesses resulting from having the chemotherapy. Cancer is a big business to cut it short. I hardly cost the NHS, which is the health body here in England, anything compared to what I would have cost them if I had gone down the chemotherapy route.

If you are given a diagnosis you just want to take any straw that gives you some hope. There is so much hype and so much fear attached to cancer. I needed a lot of self-enquiry, a lot of looking into myself, to be sure that this was really true for me that I wanted to go down the alternative route.

Initially I couldn't take in too many other peoples' stories. I was so busy with myself. I could take the story in from my friend because I knew her. I couldn't go online and research. I researched for this particular cancer that I found a forum where it seemed like people were into alternative treatment there. I said, "Look folks, I have non-Hodgkin's Lymphoma, is there anybody out there who has cured themselves in a purely natural way?"

I got nothing back and I felt really low. Then I got one short reply back from a doctor who had also signed up for this forum and she said, "Well unfortunately you are the type of person who does need chemotherapy to really get rid of the cancer." It floored me so I didn't want to hear any other people's stories.

I think doing this very clean diet really put me in touch with some very, very strong inner voice. I felt that I couldn't listen to anyone else; I just had to listen to my own truth. There came even a point where it was so vital to listen to this little voice inside me that I thought, 'Right, if that means I die eventually, well we all die eventually.' Very existential questions came up for me and to follow my own truth was more important than listening to lots of other people. My own truth was, 'No, just do it, just carry on. You don't feel bad; you are doing what you can do. You feel great really.' Yes there are these pockets of fear, at five o'clock or four o'clock in the middle of the night, when everything is dark.

Really during the day when I did my program, when I had my third green juice in the afternoon I thought, 'Wow I can take that on.'

There was a time where I said everybody has to do what I did but I almost feel that the most important thing is to really get informed and to listen to your own truth. Sometimes I think healing works best when people believe in what they are doing and it sits right with them and there is an active involvement in their healing. It's not just about lying back and receiving the chemotherapy and saying, "Oh yes, I do everything the doctor says," but that there is really some kind of conscious involvement.

I can't say that what I did is the only way. It certainly it is for me and if I would have another cancer diagnosis, really I would do and try everything I can, to get rid of it in this way again.

I did try to stay away from this seeing this tumor as having invaded my body and I that had to *kill* the tumor. I really thought, 'My body has created something and rather than killing it, what is the message? What is my body wanting to tell me?' I tried to reframe it in a more positive way. Instead of saying, "I want to kill this tumor in my breast," I worked with images and I worked with my own little fantasies that I spun around. I always tried to make it positive. For me it was really important that I somehow embrace this part of myself and say, "What's your message? What have I done to you? What can I do better? What would you like me to do?" I got such a loving sense of myself that the tumor eventually broke up into nothing.

I still go for these regular checkups. Often they send student doctors in and they try to find this tumor and it's not there...

By Nuro Weidemann

Points To Remember:

➤ Nuro's very clean diet consisted of mostly vegetables and lots of fresh green juices, three or four glasses every day.

➤ Do not make any decisions out of fear.

➤ Know that you can regain your strength and power.

➤ Nuro performed coffee enemas.

➤ She used castor oil packs over her liver to help it cleanse and renew.

➤ Meditation is always very beneficial.

➤ Sunbathe in moderation. Much research has proven the benefits of sunshine against cancer.

➤ Nuro stopped working while she was healing. Although this is not possible for everyone, what is possible for you?

➤ Create your own private spa at home and take care of yourself.

➤ Ask yourself, 'What makes me happy?' and do those things.

➤ Walk outside in the fresh air and sunshine.

➤ Recognize that tumors and cancer and other 'dis-eases' can disappear when your body is given what it needs.

➤ Make your decisions after self-enquiry. Look within and ask, 'Is this true for me? Is this what I want and need?'

➤ Do not believe what others tell you even when they present themselves with authority. There is no 'authority' over you, but yourself. This is too important to take a back seat and simply do what you are told. It is vital to listen to your own voice.

➤ Become well informed as you listen to and trust your own truth.

➤ Healing works best when people believe in what they are

doing, when it sits right with them and there is an active involvement in their own healing.

➤ Recognize that your body has created the illness. Ask your body, "What is the message you want to tell me? What have I done to you? What can I do better?"

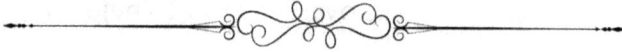

10   Healtherized Version Of The Standard Ketogenic Diet Dissolves Breast Cancer

For years patients and doctors have had very positive results using a ketogenic diet for Epilepsy. Specifically The Johns Hopkins Adult Epilepsy Center and the Johns Hopkins Ketogenic Diet Center for children have been using versions of the ketogenic diet and a modified Atkin's diet as diet therapy for Epilepsy for many, many years. As you'll hear in the story below, Meryl Streep stared in a movie depicting a true-life story about Epilepsy and the ketogenic diet used at the hospital, entitled, 'First Do No Harm.' Watch a clip at http://www.youtube.com/watch?v=DDFsLe5FbeQ. Can modifications of low carbohydrate, high fat diets, be used successfully against cancer? Elaine's amazing story shows us what is possible when the determination to heal is coupled with her modified ketogenic diet:

I created a modified version of the standard ketogenic diet, which I used to cure my breast cancer. From my research I have found that it also works to get Type 1 Diabetics off insulin. I linked cancer, epilepsy and Type 1 Diabetes together and that's how I was able to create my ketogenic diet and help myself.

I was diagnosed with invasive ductal adenocarcinoma. I was told that it was a Stage 2 cancer and it was a very strong, a Grade 3, almost 4 out of 4. I was estrogen and progesterone positive. I also had vascular invasion in and out, meaning that the cancer was probably elsewhere in my body, through my bloodstream. Two out of three lymph nodes that were removed when they did the initial lumpectomy, showed positive for cancer. I was told I needed very aggressive treatment of chemotherapy and radiation or my cancer would be in my bones and in my vital organs in no time.

After I had the x-rays and mammograms I had a lumpectomy. I had several biopsies that were positive for cancer. After my lumpectomy, the pathology confirmed all of this. I refused aggressive treatment of chemotherapy and radiation because when they said, 'aggressive', that scared me. I have seen a lot of people, some of my relatives and some of my good friends, die from cancer and the side effects of chemotherapy and radiation. Nobody was cured. I thought that if I had to go, I would not be going that way.

I had pressure from my surgeon and from my oncologist. When I refused the treatment, they were telling me they were scared for me because my cancer was very, very aggressive.

Some of my relatives were saying to me, "You can't refuse everything, you know." They were very scared that I would be dying. At first I didn't know if I would be dying or not but that's the decision that felt right with me, not to go through these treatments. I met a lady named Monique, who I was put in touch with, a little angel who was put on my road. She cured her Stage IV terminal cancer after she was given six months to live, over 14 years ago and she was my inspiration. She helped me get the guts, the back up to stand up to my doctors and to everybody else because she did it, so I figured I could do it too.

After I was diagnosed and I took my decision to not go through the chemo and radiation treatments I just felt like a ton of bricks was lifted off my shoulders and I did not have to worry about those treatments, what those treatments would do.

I was getting so much pressure from my oncologist that I had gone to the initial radiation visit and I met the doctor. The doctor was a really, really nice lady and she explained to me they would have to measure me and where my tumor was, close to my sternum bone in between my two breasts. She explained that it was close to my heart and it was close to my lungs and they would have to shoot me at an angle. I would only have minimal chances of having lung and heart damage. I never went back. That scared me. I figured that I just had a problem with cancer that was plenty enough for me and I didn't want to risk having heart problems, lung problems, not feeling my arms, being numb in my arm like some people were saying, having joint pain, losing my hair. I have good long hair, I just didn't want to lose my hair. I just thought that it was not for me and if I had to go, I would go peacefully, not that way.

About thirteen years ago, first of all, my son was diagnosed with Type 1 Diabetes and his pediatrician at the time, Dr. Go was a little angel; she saved his life. He was between life and death; he came really close. About a year after he was diagnosed with Type 1 Diabetes he became really ill. He had a high fever and he kept vomiting. For a Type 1 Diabetic they keep telling you to check ketones and ketones are bad. I was checking his urine and he had a lot of ketones so I called Dr. Go and she didn't take any chances. I went to see her with my baby, he was about three years old at the time and she decided to put him in the hospital to make sure he would not be dehydrated. When you are sick with ketones and you are diabetic, they are afraid that you will get dehydrated and you get both acidosis and ketosis which are dangerous.

When he went in the hospital, I kept checking the ketones and he kept having a lot of ketones. He was not eating because he was vomiting. He could not hold any solids and all I get him to drink was diet ginger ale. He would not even hold the water. His blood sugar started to decrease and drop and drop constantly. He was in the hospital for a couple of days. I kept decreasing his insulin dose. I kept giving him regular soda to try and bring back up his blood sugar because it kept dropping like crazy. It was amazing. By the time he got released from the hospital he was completely off insulin. For three full days after the experiment at the hospital with the high fever and a lot of ketones, it was like he was cured for three full nights and three full days. Then the ketones stopped and I was thinking, 'What happened?' because he had to be put back on insulin. I was racking my brain, I was trying to figure it out, figure out what I fed him, what I gave him, what I did that could have produced that. I was so terribly disappointed that he had to go back on insulin. I spoke to the doctor, the endocrinologist at the time and I was told that, "Often newly diagnosed patients have a honeymoon phase and sometimes before all cells go dead, the body starts working again." I kept thinking, 'There has to be a logical explanation for this.' I kept thinking, 'What did I do?'

The answer came about another year later when I saw a movie on television, just by pure chance. It was called 'First Do No Harm'. It's what the doctors swear to do when they become doctors. They swear not to harm their patients first. The movie was about the ketogenic diet from Johns Hopkins Medical Center. It's the traditional ketogenic diet that uses a combination of high fat versus low carbohydrate and low protein and the fat comes mainly from dairy, high in cream and a lot of fat from red meat.

It just clicked right when I saw that movie and then I did research about the diet and I bought the book from Dr. John Freeman. I understood what had happened to my son. When he got the high fever, he had high ketones just like the children that are put on the diet at Johns Hopkins Medical Center to treat epilepsy. It switches the body to burning fat instead of glucose so he didn't have any glucose going into his body. The glucose is a problem with Type 1 Diabetics. They have a problem processing glucose and carbohydrates. It just became all clear to me and it went the whole circle that this is what happened, so I linked Type 1 Diabetes and epilepsy through this way.

I went to Dr. Go the pediatrician again with my son and she helped us. We went on the traditional ketogenic diet; well we tried. At the time you had to fast for 48 hours before going on the diet so I fasted along with my son for 48 hours. Again I got my son completely off insulin during the fast but when I started the traditional ketogenic diet, high in dairy, 'boom' I had to put him right back on insulin, it didn't work. So I was terribly, terribly disappointed but I thought, 'There has to be a reason, there has to be a way.'

I was young at the time and I didn't know much. It took years later when I got diagnosed with my own cancer to figure things out.

First, when I was diagnosed with cancer I tried a diet with organic vegetables, the fruits and only fresh foods. I removed dairy. My cancer was very aggressive; it was just like my oncologist had said. It did not work. The cancer kept growing and I had this lump sticking out of my breast and it became really, really hard. It was like a rock. Only six months after my lumpectomy the tumor came back much bigger than the initial tumor.

While I was trying this diet that did not work for me because my cancer was too aggressive, I just happened to see online information about Dr. William B Coley back in the 1930s or 40s. This doctor was inoculating the cancer patients by injecting a toxin and he was making them have a high fever and 'boom' the patients would just get cured because the fever, the toxin would get them sick. Sometimes they would vomit too. I started researching on this because I thought, 'Oh my God, this is too much of a coincidence.'

This could not be just a coincidence. It was the same scenario as with my son. He gets sick, he gets a high fever and he is cured! Dr. Coley's patients get sick with the toxin that he produces the disease with, they get high fever and then they get cured. So I started researching about this and sure enough the patients in his case study who were getting so sick, were not eating. Fever is an appetite suppressor so in the case study over and over again; starvation was mentioned in the best cases of remission of cancer. In Dr. Coley's patient case studies, the people who were cured, with the best cases of remission and the quickest, were involved with starvation. They were so sick they had vomiting and anorexia. Some of them couldn't eat because they had large tumors in their throat and starvation kept coming up again and again.

Again, starvation is linked to ketones. When you don't eat you have ketones in your urine and you switch to burning fat instead of glucose. Everything was being linked again with cancer to the ketogenic diet. I started researching the case studies from Dr. Coley, about the ones who were fed and what kind of diet they were fed. I could not find anything because there is no information about their diets except for starvation.

I came across Dr. Gerson. When his diet alone was not working for very advanced patients, such as very advanced cancer or gastric cancer, he experimented by adding the toxin from Dr. Coley's research, to his patients' protocol along with his diet. With Dr. Gerson there is a very detailed diet so I could see that the diet was free of all the major allergens for at least six to eight weeks. This information encouraged me to create my own ketogenic diet, free from all major allergens, meaning: dairy, soy, all the grains including wheat and fructose and glucose.

I used my ketogenic diet on myself and my cancer was gone after two weeks. I went to my oncologist. I had started my diet for three or four days and my lump was the size of a small egg. It was all hard and he looked at me, I'll never forget his face, I'll always remember. His face was so serious and he said, "I'm taking this very seriously. This is a reoccurrence. It's coming back in the same area as your lumpectomy. It's because you refused radiation that it's coming back in the same area. You need to go to the surgeon as soon as possible." Again he repeated to me, "I'm taking this very seriously." He wanted me to have surgery as soon as possible. I was not even out of the oncologist's office parking lot when I had the surgeon's office calling me for an appointment for the next business day. The first time I was rushed into having all these tests done and the lumpectomy within one week of diagnosis. I decided I was not going to be rushed. I just started my ketogenic diet. I had just started to switch my body from burning the fat instead of the sugar. I wanted to give it time to work so I postponed the appointment at the surgeon's office. By the time I went to see my surgeon, the lump went from the size of a small egg to about the size of a chick pea but more oval, still like the shape of an egg.

My oncologist had sent a report to the surgeon's office. He had put the size of the tumor in the report and the surgeon did the sonogram. My sonogram showed that whatever was left there was not cancer. She did a biopsy and the biopsy later came back negative. She thought that the oncologist had made a mistake because he put the size of the tumor in the report and she was seeing something much smaller, in very little time.

After everything came back negative and my surgeon sent back the report to the oncologist, the oncologist's office was calling me because they wanted me to go for more tests and a mammogram. They didn't believe that there was nothing there.

Then I tried my diet on my son and sure enough it worked. Without all the allergens, my son, for a whole week, was able to eat and drink as much as he wanted without any calorie restriction and no need for any insulin. He is only fifteen and the diet for him was very, very difficult. He was starting school and he didn't want to bring his lunch so he got off the diet. He has trouble believing that this is a possible cure because he has been brainwashed that there is no cure for Type 1 Diabetes and I'm just his mom.

Based on my son's experience when he was little and having problems with dairy, I tried soy. Soy did the same thing and Dr. Go told me if they have an internal reaction, an allergy or intolerance to dairy, a lot of her patients also react the same way to soy. I did not take any chances. I tried to make my diet as foolproof as I could by removing all the major allergens and anything else that is known to cause a reaction in the body. For example, for me when I eat tomatoes and I eat too much, I have a rash like eczema, so I didn't eat any of that either. I tried to mimic when you fast and you don't eat, you have nothing that can impact your body negatively or cause an autoimmune reaction inside that you don't visually see.

In my research I came across Dr. Otto Warburg. He won a Nobel Prize in Medicine and basically he says that sugar fuels cancer, that's the primary cause of cancer. He says when the cancer feeds on sugar it causes a by-product of lactic acid and the lactic acid causes the pH to become more acidic and the more acidic, the more aggressive the cancer is, as per research.

I also looked at the sources of lactic acid because if I have cancer and I have a problem with lactic acid, I don't want to add more lactic acid in my diet. I found that lactic acid comes from dairy products, bread, beer and other products. Those are some of the reasons why I removed dairy from my diet but also because dairy is an allergen and there is a lot of research that shows dairy is linked to several diseases including Type 1 Diabetes, cancer, multiple sclerosis, Parkinson's disease and several others. Dairy was removed for all these reasons.

Gilli gave me a testimony after using my diet. She had a lumpectomy, just like me and after she refused chemotherapy and radiation the cancer came back, in both breasts. She had three tumors. On my diet, after a month, two of the tumors were gone. The third one was gone after the second month on my diet. Gilli was the one who helped me and pushed me to write the book.

I show the parallel with hundreds of autoimmune diseases because they all have inflammation in common. I targeted my diet to boost glutathione and to be anti-inflammatory. There are other people who are healing themselves on my diet, every day. The people I have helped are also helping other people and it's starting to be a domino effect.

This is my diet of hope, my diet that comes from my heart, my own research. I lived it and I know what its like. I hope it can help others.

My book is called *The Cantin Ketogenic Diet for Cancer, Type 1 Diabetes and Other Ailments*. In the book you will find the diet, how to do the diet, recipes, and examples of things to eat. My diet is also Vegan friendly and that's a first with the ketogenic diet. My book is green. I picked the color green for the color of life, the trees, the plants and also the color of hope.

By Elaine Cantin

Update: April 2013
Elaine wanted you to know that she is battling breast cancer for a third time. After working 60 hours a week and almost losing her mother, the stress has caused a reoccurrence of Elaine's breast cancer. This new tumor has reoccurred very close to the original tumor. Recently her oncologist told Elaine that her Stage IV cancer 'must' be throughout her body and that she should have listened to their recommendations and taken chemotherapy and radiation.

Update: June 2013
Great news – scans and tests show that there is no cancer elsewhere in her body. With Elaine back on her modified ketogenic diet and reducing her working hours and stress levels, she is back on track and the tumor is shrinking again. Now tests on the tumor show that there is no cancer there.

This addition to Elaine's healing journey shows us that we must reduce stress and take care of ourselves, in order to stay healthy and cancer-free.

Points To Remember:

> Make the decisions that feel right to you.

> If others can do it, so can you.

> Ketosis: When your body switches to burning fat for fuel because there is no glucose available.

> You can measure ketones in the urine with ketone strips.

> A starvation diet will produce ketones.

> If there is no sugar in the blood from starvation, a diabetic's need for insulin injections will diminish. In Elaine's son, when he got sick and couldn't eat, his need for insulin was 0%.

> The traditional ketogenic diet used at Johns Hopkins Medical Center uses a combination of high fat versus low carbohydrate and low protein. This diet allows high fat pasteurized dairy products, dairy cream and cooked saturated fat from meat, which are acid forming and congesting. Dairy products contain lactose, a form of sugar.

> Type 1 Diabetics have trouble processing glucose and carbohydrates.

> In Dr. Coley's patient case studies, the people who were cured the fastest, with the best cases of remission, were involved with starvation; whether they were so sick they had vomiting and anorexia or they couldn't eat because they had large tumors in their throat.

> Elaine's diet is a modified version of the standard ketogenic diet, which has removed all processed and allergenic foods. It removes all the major allergens: soy, dairy, all grains including wheat, fructose and glucose. It is

designed to be anti-inflammatory and to boost glutathione, a most important antioxidant for detoxification.

➤ When Elaine tweaked the ketogenic diet with her own modifications her aggressive cancer was gone after only two weeks.

➤ Dr. Otto Warburg, Nobel Prize in Medicine: "Sugar fuels and is the primary cause of cancer. When cancer feeds on sugar it creates lactic acid, which increases blood pH, causing more aggressive cancers."

➤ If you have a reoccurrence get right back on track and don't let it cause you to do something you might regret later.

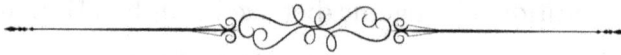

11 From Cancerous Liposarcoma To Self Healing With Trust And Conviction

I had a very small lump in my right thigh for about seven or eight years. I went to the doctors twice and they told me, "It's no big deal. It's fat tissue." I am very small so I thought, 'That doesn't make sense,' but both doctors told me the same thing. Then during Christmas of 2010, my daughter said, "Mom, your leg looks kind of funny. It looks like the bump is coming out." So I went to a doctor. The first doctor was not available. I had to go back for a second time. Then I had to go for a third time.

By the third appointment I was already looking into what it could be in my leg and I found out from Google that it could be a Lipoma, which is fat tissue. I made a printout. I went to see an internist and he said to me, "It's no big deal, it's just fat tissue."

I said, "It doesn't hurt but it's bothering me when I sit down now."

The funny thing is that he printed the same thing from Google that I had printed the night before. He said, "Okay, I will send you to a one-day surgery."

I agreed and went to a one-day surgery. They didn't measure it. They didn't say anything. They were very casual. I had the surgery then I went home. I had a very big cut and I was open horizontally which later I learned is totally wrong; because of the muscle, they have to do surgery the opposite way. So I went home and by

Monday or Tuesday the surgeon called me and said, "Ten percent of the cells in the tumor that I removed were cancer cells. You need to go immediately to see an Orthopedic Surgeon and an Oncologist."

I panicked and called my brother. I only have a brother here and I am from Honduras originally. He said, "We are going to do whatever we have to."

I went to my best friend and she was crying because her sister had just died of cancer not too long ago and so now to hear that I had it was just devastating for her.

I went to see a doctor at the University of Minnesota. He's a top specialist in the state for treating liposarcomas on legs and arms. He had me see his intern. I saw his intern for about 45 minutes. A friend of mine, another oncologist and my brother were present. The specialist came in and he said to me, "We will just do surgery. You will have to do some radiation and then you'll do surgery again."

I asked if there was anything else and he just kind of brushed me off and didn't say very much. I said, "You haven't done any tests. You haven't asked me much about my history."

He said, "I know about these kinds of things." He didn't want to hear anything I had to say. I did not like him at all to start with because he just didn't want to hear anything.

After that I went home and I really started to worry because it began to sink in that I had cancer. I really had a gut feeling that something was not right with what the doctor was telling me. I started reading on the Internet and in books and I did so much research, tons of research. I even think I crossed www.IncredibleHealingJournals.com at one point. I started reading everything available, whether from professionals, universities and people. I signed into two or three Yahoo groups. I looked at everything I could. I asked everybody. Within days of seeing the first oncologist, I felt that I just couldn't go on with radiation.

Then my brother insisted that we go see a different doctor for another opinion. We went to Mayo and there was a very nice oncologist there but he also had the same recipe, "You've got to do radiation for six weeks and if you don't do it, it's going to spread. You have to do it now. You have no time."

He was pressing me a lot but he was at least willing to listen to what I had to say and I kept asking, "Do you have any alternatives?"

By then I had already read a lot of stuff and he said, "No we don't have any statistics that alternative medicine works. I can send you to have massage therapy or yoga if you wish." That's all he could offer.

I agreed to come and see him again in six months and I said, "I'm not going to do what you are recommending because I feel like I can do other things. There has to be other ways. I could see he was thinking, 'She's crazy.'

Then he brought in an orthopedic surgeon and they were already planning to schedule me for surgery even though I had not agreed to it. I told them, "No," and I sat there and they had to bring a patient advocate because I was so adamant, "No I'm not going to do it, no I'm not going to do it."

He had me sign something and I said, "I'll sign whatever you want. I'm just telling you I am going to use you for diagnostics but I am not going to do what you are recommending to me."

My brother was kind of scared and he said, "Well you need to put it in the balance of what it is, the impact that it is going to have."

I said, "No this is my life" and I was very adamant. I almost kicked him out of the room. I said, "No, I'm going to do at this point what I feel is right for me."

It took going to see the second oncologist, then going to a third one to really reaffirm that I had to follow my heart, that I just had to follow my gut, my instinct, my body. By then I had already tried the Macrobiotics Diet. I had read the Budwig Diet. I had read the Raw Diet and the Gerson Therapy. I tried each diet for a couple of months.

They took the lump, thinking that it was non-malignant but by December it came back. I hadn't gone to see the oncologist but I noticed that when I got stressed in December it got very big. I started thinking this for me was a wake up call and I needed to deal with a lot of emotional stuff.

I decided to start working on forgiveness. I had issues with my parents. I hadn't talked to them in a long time. It took me almost three months to write them a letter but I did. I noticed when I wrote that letter the lump got reduced by about half an inch and I measured it; so then I understood it was not only food. As far as food goes, at the beginning I was doing some organic but not everything. Now I am doing everything organic because I realize everything that goes into my mouth goes into my body.

Still, I had to get very serious about food so it was about that time when I found out about Elaine. Somebody in the Yahoo group had mentioned her name and that she had a group in Facebook. Her diet made sense to me a lot because it seemed balanced.

I noticed when I started her diet with forgiveness, that's when my lump began to reduce itself. It was just the beginning. I had to dig deep, deep, deep. It's a journey because I'm still doing that. I changed a lot of things.

I had begun doing a lot of forgiveness work with friends. I understood I also needed to do a lot of forgiveness work with myself because I wasn't doing that. That was yet another part of the journey, a very, very tender and harsh part, with a lot of spiritual work. By then I had skipped my MRI because I was not ready to do it. A year went by and I hadn't had the MRI. They would keep telling me, "Come here, you have to do the MRI."

I went back to Mayo and I told them, "I will have the MRI but I don't want to have the ink put on me, the chemical. The doctor was not happy about it and I asked, "Is there another way to look at my lump? Can you do different scanning?"

He said, "Nope, we have to do it this way."

I went ahead and did the MRI but I didn't take the liquid with me so they were not happy about it. They wanted me to sign some releases. They wanted to study the lump because they didn't have many people my age with that type of cancer. I told them I wasn't there to be a research person for them. I had to sign and I didn't want to and I said, "I don't feel hurt by this hospital so I'm not going to sign anything."

I just did my MRI. The second time when I saw the doctor I said, "It's been a year. I know there is oxygen therapy." I mentioned Gerson. I mentioned everything I knew by then and he totally laughed. He laughed at me. I was very disappointed because I really liked this doctor and I thought, 'Well he doesn't have to do everything but at least he can show that he cares a little bit.'

He told me, "We have no numbers that prove that any alternative treatment helps cancer."

I almost cried in front of him and I said, "I'm just not coming back."

He told me, "If you don't come back and if you don't have surgery you are going to have this spread within a year and we are not going to be able to do anything for you."

I said, "That's fine. That's the road I'm willing to take," and I walked out of Mayo. I didn't let them photograph my leg because they wanted to photograph it for their research so I just said, "No," and I never went back.

I became so frustrated with the medical community. I think I was stressed, not about the cancer but stressed dealing with the medical system. I feel that their agenda was to do surgery, chemotherapy or radiation no matter what I said. Every time I entered a room it was the lump, it was not me; it was a lump that they needed to take from my body. They didn't see me. They never asked me if there was anything going on in my house. Was I stressed? How was my nutrition? They never took any blood tests. Mayo did at the end, only when I demanded.

After being so frustrated one day, I posted on Facebook that I was appalled because in the document Mayo handed me at my second appointment, on the first line after your name is, 'Do you have a will?' I got so infuriated by this and I said, "I'm not dying." I understand there is a reason behind it but they could at least put it on the last line. I thought, 'They have an agenda. You're going to die. You have cancer. You're going to die, that's it.' I became so harsh with the hospitals and the nurses and everyone else. Many times I went and apologized and said, "It's not your fault. It's the system but this is no way to treat people." I just felt everything was set up for you to fail, to accept nothing but radiation, chemotherapy and surgery. They are the experts and they are not willing to hear about anything. After posting that on Facebook a friend of mine who is a Social Worker at a different hospital in Minneapolis said, "Evangelina you should try this hospital. They have a clinic and they are very patient orientated."

By then I was on Elaine's diet and I noticed there were a lot of things changing with me, emotionally, physically and spiritually. I was in a different place. For a year I was studying until two or three in the morning on the Internet, figuring out what to do. I had been gardening. I started changing my lifestyle; when I say lifestyle I mean everything, everything. From the time I get up until the time I go to bed, how I brush my teeth, how I'm thankful for things in my life, how I cook, how I treat others. I just became very observant of everything. I felt that everything had a place in that lump that I had.

I went to see yet a fourth doctor, an orthopedic surgeon and oncologist and he told me the same thing although he was very nice, he was very caring, he held my hand.

He said, "Evangelina if you don't do anything you're going to have this spread."

I said, "I know that."

He said, "Why did you come to see me?" and I said, "Because you are a doctor and you took an oath and I think you should help me." I just said it to him, "You're a doctor. You can order oxygen therapy. You can order Vitamin C IV for me."

He said, "No I can't. That doesn't work. We don't do that here."

I said, "Yes you can. Why do I have to go outside of the country?"

He said, "We know of a doctor who does alternative medicine, maybe I can make a phone call for you but I'm telling you this, you are just going to the wrong place." He said, "I want you to go for an MRI because you haven't had an MRI with the liquid."

I said, "I will do it only if you promise me you will help me after. Either sending me to someone for an IV of Vitamin C or some alternative."

He said, "Okay, I will try to help you."

So I did the MRI. This time I was ready. I thought they were going to poison me so I prepared two or three days before by taking a lot of herbs. I ate a lot of Cilantro and did a lot of juicing. I also did a lot of spiritual preparation. I went and did the MRI and the interesting thing is that when I was inside the machine, I closed my eyes and prayed and the whole time I saw this purple light. Later I learned this is one of the Chakras. It is in the top of your head and is the color purple. That was the only thing I was seeing with my eyes closed which was very interesting. I waited. Within three or four days I was thinking, 'Why are they not calling?' I got worried but in my heart and in my gut I knew everything was okay.

The orthopedic surgeon had told me, "Evangelina we have to cut your leg. Otherwise this is just going to spread any time now."

Finally, I got a call from his nurse saying, "Evangelina, the doctor has received the results and there is no evidence of metastatic disease and the nodules you have are so low density we cannot distinguish what it is."

The doctor didn't call me. He had scheduled surgery without my permission but he never called me back again.

I knew then, even if I had a little bit, I had to follow my gut. I had to follow my body, now more so than ever. I strongly decided, 'Okay, what I'm doing is working. I know that I have a purpose.' I always thought from day one that this was a blessing for me. I know it sounds weird but I feel like its changing the ways I can help other people and help my own family and spread the word that there are other ways to do this.

It's not about how long you live it's about how good a life you do have when you serve and you are here for a purpose.

A lot of the supplements I used, I figured out first by reading about what my cells needed and what my body needed because I know my body better than anybody. I had to figure out what to take and

I learned to listen to my body. Sometimes I went to the health store and suddenly I just found something that caught my attention so I would buy it. I didn't know what it was for and I would get home, do a search and sure enough it was something specifically for repair of the cells, for tissue repair or for the immune system. It was like the universe, or God or whatever you believe in, gives you all these things and if you listen really, truly, your body helps you heal.

For me it has been a complete journey, a holistic journey because I see it as doing emotional work on my own, doing forgiveness work and learning to love myself. I have changed how I eat. I have changed my routine. It's a lot of work, a lot, but I want to live and I know there is another way than putting chemo or poison in my body.

I found a doctor who believes in alternative medicine and he did a lot of testing lately and everything is normal. He was very pleased because nothing in my immune system shows that I am deficient. In fact he was quite surprised that everything is working. Every blood test he took, the natural killer cells, everything came back absolutely normal.

I am healthy, extremely healthy. I am doing a lot of meditation.

I found a group where a lot of people who are being treated for cancer take a lot of classes for free and I am participating by writing and cooking, with the goal of eventually volunteering to help others.

I am doing what I can, where I am with my own healing. It's a journey and you have to be very, very dedicated. It's not a Band-Aid. It's a change of lifestyle. It's not just for one day. It's a total change and it's ongoing daily. You check yourself every day, 'How am I doing in this part? What can I do better? What should I do now?' while following your heart, your gut and your body.

I had a sister who had a brain tumor. She didn't die of that at the age of 16, she died of something else but I knew that she was very damaged by the chemotherapy. From seeing so many people die, I just thought, 'Well it doesn't help anybody. It extends life for maybe two, five years at the most. Most people lose their hair and that's not natural. How can that be natural?'

I grew up in Honduras and we do believe a lot in witches and good witches and we believe a lot in nature, herbs, healers and shamans. I felt those things could work, plants and nature. That's what they are here for.

I've seen people who have cancer and they just survive two years and then they are gone. I just had this feeling inside. Every time he mentioned radiation I had this sort of knot in my stomach and I thought that's not a normal reaction, that's when you have conflict. I thought there has to be something to it but now they have my results. "Look! Look! You told me it was going to be in my lungs." They don't even find anything in my lungs, nothing.

The lump on my leg is still smaller and I have been using 'salve' a little bit too. Last summer I didn't touch it and it was fine but I still have a little bit of it and I don't know if this is scar tissue or if it's a mix in how I see it. I'm forty-five now. It took probably ten years to show up in my body so it's going to take some time to heal. To me it has become like a meter. When I get angry or have any stress I notice that the lump will hurt, just as an indicator. It's like the lump says, "'Okay you are doing something that is not helpful. It's not good spiritually. It's not good for your body. It's not good as a stressor. You can do better."

I was thinking it took time to grow, it's going to take some time also for me to really be complete because I'm healing, emotionally and spiritually. I'm finding out what I want to do in life, which might be to help others through my experience, I don't know.

It is a very holistic thing. It's changing everything. I feel like it's all going together, one thing, the next thing; I do one step then I have to do the next step, until it's complete.

So it's still there somewhat and I'm treating it with the black salve. That's a very painful thing to do and I did it twice already and the first time that I did it you could see the little thing that came out, one of the roots. They told me the nodules were small so that was probably one of the small lumps I still have there.

I put it on this weekend and I can tell you that it's so swollen and it's so red that yesterday I stayed home because its hard for me to drive or to sit down. I have to be very careful. At the same time the immune system is responding to it. After you are done and it has come out, it closes right after. It closes like nothing. It doesn't disturb any other tissues. It's amazing what nature does.

When they did the surgery, they thought it was non-malignant. Number one, they totally did it in the wrong way because that's not how you cut the leg, you cut it vertically and he left such a huge scar. It's ugly. It's very ugly. With these things you don't have all that.

When he opened my leg he touched my nerves and he told me, "It's going to take two years before you can feel your nerve again in your leg." I decided to go to acupuncture. This acupuncturist is a wonderful Chinese woman. I felt my leg within two weeks of her treatment of acupuncture.

I did see her for a while to help me with stress. She had given me some bitter herbs that the Chinese use to treat cancer with. She is just wonderful. I told her mine is very rare and that's why it has to be attacked from many ways. That's why I tried everything I could.

I have this wonderful doctor who has sent me to biofeedback and has me doing a lot of yoga and meditation. He is a medical doctor and he is a strong believer but he can't say a lot either. He is in the minority right now but he does work with a wonderful team and he does know that nutrition works. I have given them Elaine's name and they are all interested about what else is working because they pass it to other patients.

More and more people are now are going this way. It's everywhere now. Everyone wants to know what should I take, what should I eat and I always keep saying food is so important.

Heal yourself by loving, love, love, self-love.

By Evangelina Aguilar

Points To Remember:

- Take a friend or family member with you to appointments. They help keep you calm and remember what to ask as well as what was said.

- This is your life. You have to do what feels right for you.

- Follow your heart. Follow your gut, your instinct. Follow your body.

- Try different diets and therapies until you find what suits you best.

- Everything that goes into your mouth goes into your body.

- Get serious about food.

- Healing is a complete and holistic journey.

- Do forgiveness work with yourself and others. Dig deep.

- Healing is more than nutrition. Healing involves your spiritual and emotional bodies as well as your physical and mental bodies.

- You have the right to be treated with respect. You have a choice to deal with those who respect you and your wishes. You also have the right to refuse treatment from those who do not respect you and your wishes.

- Do the things that please you most.

- Recognize that everything has a place in your 'ill-ness'.

- Cancer can be a blessing in disguise.

- It's not about how long you live it's about how good a life you do have when you serve and you are here for a purpose.

- Find a doctor who believes in alternative therapies and nutrition. Have him test you to be sure you are not deficient in nutrients.

- Meditate.
- Do what you can, where you are with your own healing.
- Be very, very dedicated to healing yourself.
- When you get the feeling, that knot in your stomach, your body is notifying you of a conflict with your best interest. Take heed.
- Sometimes a tumor will flare up in pain, or you may have another recognizable symptom. This can be interpreted as an indicator from your body that what you are doing is not in line with healing.
- Heal yourself by loving you. Practice self-love.

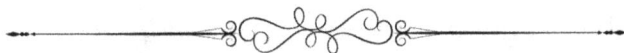

12   What Is Possible For You?

I hope these stories have inspired you with hope and practical knowledge so you may apply what rings true and heal your life.

The path of healing is a wondrous adventure strewn with obstacles that will test your resolve and prove your resilience.

Even when people are told they will surely die, they have brought themselves back from the brink of death. They have moved forward through illness, to live healthy, happy and fulfilling lives.

These remarkable stories are not few and far between. Every day, more and more people are finding their own way to healing.

For some people, cancer is one of life's greatest gifts.

I wish this for you.

With much love and hope for the future,

Lisa

oxo

Thank You!

Thank you for buying this book and trusting me to offer valuable information. I sincerely hope you use the information in this book to help your body heal.

I would be thrilled to hear how you have used the concepts in this or any of my books. You are welcome to send your comments to support@thegoodwitch.ca or use the contact form at www.thegoodwitch.ca/contact.

Please visit my website at www.thegoodwitch.ca where you will find more tools and tips for healing yourself.

You may wish to visit www.incrediblehealingjournals.com to see videos of these and many other remarkable stories, where people share the best ideas, principles and methods they use to heal.

If you would like to learn the practical steps to healing as taught in the '10 Key Principles Of Healing Transformational Experience', visit www.HealingCancer.ca.

Until next time,
Happy Healing!
Lisa

The Favor Of A Review

Reviews, ratings and comments about this book are whole-heartedly appreciated. If you have enjoyed this visit into the world of healing cancer, you can leave a review by visiting this book's page on Amazon or Barnes & Noble.

You'll also have a chance to rate the book and share your rating with your friends on Facebook and Twitter, after you turn the last page if this is a Kindle book.

I read every review of my books and love to hear what readers have to say. It guides me to write books that are more likely to help others. If you have a moment, I'd be grateful for your time.

Thank You, Thank You, Thank You!

Connect With The Authors

Some authors prefer not to be contacted and we have not been given permission to share their contact information.

Connect With Linda Devine

As a Success and Wellness Coach Linda helps women reach their full potential as individuals. Her focus is on helping women with critical illnesses such as breast cancer, to get their life back. When we are faced with these types of challenges we are often scared, confused and feel out of control. We want to make the right choices but are not sure how or where to turn. As a holistic coach, Linda has been through this transformational change and knows firsthand what it is like to be diagnosed with breast cancer. Together with Linda you will go through the process of looking at all your options objectively, making positive, healthy changes and ensuring that you make the right choices for yourself.

Linda's Website: www.lindadevine.com

Linda on LinkedIn: www.linkedin.com/in/lindadevine

Pattie McDonald

See Pattie's story complete with shocking before and after photographs here: www.incrediblehealingjournals.com/an-incredible-story-breast-cancer-cured-with-escharotic/

Connect With Brenda Cobb

Brenda is the Founder and Director of The Living Foods Institute. She has an Honorary Cultural Doctorate, Therapeutic Philosophy from World University. Her mission is to teach as many people as possible how to restore and maintain their most optimum health by eating organic raw and living foods, by using detoxification and by using emotional healing work. She is recognized as a foremost leader, healer and teacher in the raw and living foods movement. Many thousands of people have taken her classes, workshops and seminars and their testimonies are awe-inspiring. People come from all over the world to Brenda's healing institute in Alabama, U.S.

Connect with Brenda and watch her video interview here: www.incrediblehealingjournals.com/ihj-interviews-brenda-cobb-on-curing-breast-cancer-and-cervical-cancer/
Brenda's Website: www.LivingFoodsInstitute.com
Brenda's Email: brenda@livingfoodsinstitute.com
Call Living Foods Institute: 800-844-9876

Connect With Kapil Arn

Kapil is presently living in New Zealand. Kapil is a Holistic Wellness Coach and is passionate about helping you to have more abundance in both your physical and financial health. Kapil's mantra is, 'Win-win-win, no losers.'

Connect with Kapil and watch his video interview here: www.incrediblehealingjournals.com/ihj-interviews-kapil-arn-on-curing-non-hodgkins-sub-cutaneous-t-cell-lymphoma/
Kapil on LinkedIn: www.nz.linkedin.com/in/kapilarn
Kapil on Facebook: www.facebook.com/kapil.arn1

Connect With Dr. Sue Gelder, ND, BSc (Hons) BioMed, BSc (Hons) Hom, FCTP, BFRP, IIHHT, TAT

Dr. Sue is a Consultant Naturopath and Author of *How I Cured My Tumor Naturally and How You May Help Cure Yours Too*. She is Managing Director at Edenique Complementary Healthcare and Entrepeneur.

Connect with Dr. Sue and watch her video interview here:
www.incrediblehealingjournals.com/ihj-interviews-dr-sue-gelder-on-curing-herself-of-an-inoperable-spinal-tumour/
Dr. Sue on LinkedIn: www.uk.linkedin.com/pub/sue-gelder/20/98a/927
Dr. Sue on Facebook: www.facebook.com/sue.gelder.5

Connect With Yvonne Chamberlain

Yvonne is a cancer survivor, Life Coach, Life Enricher and Author. She is an Independent Licensed Consultant for Life Success Consulting.
Connect With Yvonne Chamberlain and hear her audio interview:
www.incrediblehealingjournals.com/yvonne-cures-malignant-melanoma/
Yvonne's website: www.myfreedom.net.au/

Connect With Chris Wark

Chris is a passionate speaker and blogger who shares information about how to heal from cancer in a knowledgeable and smart way. More and more people are choosing a 'take charge' approach to dealing with cancer and refusing to poison their bodies with toxic drugs and radiation. They are choosing instead, like Chris ... with conviction and strength, to research their options thoroughly and to choose only those therapies that are kind and healing to their bodies. Chris shares a wealth of information on healing from cancer at his blog.

Connect with Chris and watch his video interview here: www.incrediblehealingjournals.com/chris-wark-uses-surgery-in-combination-with-holistic-raw-nutrition-to-cure-colon-cancer/ Chris's website: www.ChrisBeatCancer.com

Nuro Weidemann

Watch Nuro's video interview here: www.incrediblehealingjournals.com/incredible-healing-journals-presents-nuro-weidemann-on-curing-non-hodgkins-lymphoma/

Connect With Elaine Cantin

Elaine works tirelessly at her Facebook page sharing information about healing from all types of disease. She has extensive knowledge about using a ketogenic diet in healing cancer, epilepsy and diabetes. Connect with Elaine and the people in her Facebook Group who are using her modified ketogenic diet to heal themselves.

Connect with Elaine, learn more about her book and watch her video interview here: www.incrediblehealingjournals.com/elaine-cantin-on-how-to-cure-breast-cancer-with-her-modified-ketogenic-diet/
Elaine's Alternative Tips for Cancer, Type 1 Diabetes & Other

Ailments on Facebook:
www.facebook.com/groups/ElaineAlternativeHealthTips/

Evangelina Aguilar

Watch Evangelina's video interview here:
www.incrediblehealingjournals.com/evangelina-aguilar-shares-a-profound-journey-of-healing-from-liposarcoma/

Connect with Lisa Robbins

Lisa is a Registered Holistic Nutritionist with a Bachelor of Science in Holistic Nutrition and a certified Adult Teacher/Trainer. Teaching is her passion. Lisa has dedicated her life to transforming harmful beliefs about illness. She teaches you to become the leader in your life, to adopt a safe and health-promoting environment, without harmful experiences and to feeel your way back to health. She delivers these powerful healing messages through a varied medium of writing, audio, video and through sharing real life stories and experiences.

Free Teaching, Cleanses, Recipes: www.TheGoodWitch.ca
Videos: Watch more healing stories here:
www.IncredibleHealingJournals.com
Course: 10 Key Principles of Healing Transformational Experience at www.HealingCancer.ca
Lisa's Email: lisa@thegoodwitch.ca

Visit Us On The Web

Our Websites

www.TheGoodWitch.ca

Delicious healing recipes, tips, information and connection to hundreds of unbiased resources for healing: studies, journal articles, resource databases, books, audios and videos, many free. Recipes, cleanses, articles, interviews and free downloads are available.

www.IncredibleHealingJournals.com

The Incredible Healing Journals ~ a truly alternative healing community ~ find incredible stories of natural healing streaming through our front page. Connect with natural healers and their own stories of healing with tips, advice and support.

www.HealingCancer.ca

Home Study Course:

10 Key Principles of Healing Transformational Experience

All about Healing ~ resources, lessons, interviews, videos, audios, incredible healing stories, articles and truth!

Connect with us on Social Networks

YouTube

www.youtube.com/user/thegoodwitchca

Facebook

Incredible Healing Journals Community Group:

www.facebook.com/groups/incrediblehealingjournals/

Incredible Healing Journals Page:

www.facebook.com/IncredibleHealingJournals

The Good Witch Page: www.facebook.com/goodwitch.ca

LinkedIn

www.ca.linkedin.com/in/thegoodwitch/

Twitter

www.twitter.com/thegoodwitchca

The Cancer Journal Heal Yourself! by Lisa Robbins

A how to book with complete instructions on healing yourself –
with colourful photographs, detailed directions and connection to
hundreds of essential resources including delicious healing
recipes, key studies and journal articles, incredible healing stories,
videos, audios and much, much more. Here's what you'll find
inside:

- ➤ Expert Nutrition Advice, Tips and Warnings
- ➤ Know precisely which foods to eat more of and which foods
  to eat less of, to cleanse, nourish, heal and rebuild your
  body, its tissues, fluids and organs.
- ➤ Learn and understand exactly how to make your own
  powerful cancer fighting medicines in your own kitchen.
- ➤ Understand the 10 Key Principles of Healing and know
  how to apply these simple principles to your own life right
  now, to heal your body.
- ➤ Recipes for Amazing Herbal Medicines Proven to Kill
  Cancer
- ➤ See exactly what other people have done to cure cancer
  themselves and know exactly how you can do the same.
- ➤ Clear action steps so you can stay focused on healing.
- ➤ Gain a powerful understanding of exactly how to heal
  yourself no matter what place you are in at this moment.
- ➤ Empowering Information That Will Change Your Beliefs
  About Cancer Forever

Available in Printed and Kindle Format at:

www.Amazon.com

www.BarnesAndNoble.com

Available in instant downloadable PDF Format at:

www.TheGoodWitch.ca

www.ingramcontent.com/pod-product-compliance
Lightning Source LLC
Chambersburg PA
CBHW062057270326
41931CB00013B/3121